DR. SEBI ALKALINE DIET

The ultimate guide to dr. Sebi diet.

Approved herbs and recipes for a perfect colon, skin, and liver cleaning.

Detox your body, lose weight with energy, live healthily

TASHA DIXON

TABLE OF CONTENTS

BOOK PREFACE

I would like to dedicate this book to the great work of dr. Sebi, who at a difficult time in my life took me by the hand and guided me towards an unexpected rebirth.

His immense work inspired me to change my diet, which, at that time, was literally killing me.

when I was prey to the most destructive food addictions, I felt like I was broken inside, useless, unable to rebuild my life. In addition, the worst part was that I didn't think I could change a thing! Clumsy, heavy, without energy, and with a look that really needed changing... However, that I didn't have the courage to change. I didn't like anything about myself, and I thought my life had nothing else in store for me. Then one day I "stumbled" upon a book... Moreover, that book entered my life, my home, and my kitchen. That's when my life changed. By throwing away toxic food, i threw away what was toxic in my life, watching myself be reborn every day. Dr. Sebi, you will never know that you saved me, but I do. In addition, this is my tribute to your wonderful work.

INTRODUCTION

Dr. Sebi's alkaline diet is reputed to healing different kinds of diseases and keeping the body healthy. It is a high-fiber and low-fat diet, with a good protein content. It is rich in alkaline foods that help heal diseases and keep the body healthy. The alkaline food diet also helps with weight loss, increased energy levels, increased mental function and clarity, lower cholesterol levels and blood pressure. A balanced pH diet consists of vegetable-based foods such as vegetables, grains, fruits & some legumes.

Dr. Sebi's diet has its core in maintaining and improving health or wellness by returning the body to its original alkaline state. It is a core element of his therapeutic approach. It focuses on optimizing the body's ability to eliminate toxins. By following this diet, one can reduce one chance of getting sick. It uses familiar foods that have been proven beneficial in health care products to treat diseases such as heart disease, cancer, diabetes, and arthritis.

According to Dr. Sebi, illness and disease are a result of acidification and survive only because of the mucus, that creates an acid environment. The alkaline diet is designed to create an inhospitable environment for disease organisms and enables the body's immune system to restore and repair itself. Eating too much meat and other animal-origin products and too many processed foods is very acid-forming in the body.

Dr. Sebi suggests that by eating a predominantly plant-based alkaline food diet, we will be healthier. While occasionally eating meat, fish or poultry will not kill you, it's not good to let it become a regular habit.

Dr. Sebi's alkaline foods are important to the body's health and well-being because they return the body to its natural pH. The idea is to return blood pH levels to a point above 7.35, which will help reduce the risk of degenerative diseases and keep your body functioning at its optimal levels.

In Dr. Sebi's opinion, our body needs always be in an alkaline environment to remain healthy and effectively carry out its functions. The body has a very delicate balance between acid and alkaline and requires a slightly acidic environment. It was "designed" alkaline, but can also function in a slightly acidic environment. Maintaining a slight acidity helps the body eliminate toxins, lubricates joints, supports the immune system, and regulates blood pressure levels.

On the other hand, it also needs to be in an alkaline environment to eliminate waste from the body. The alkaline diet is designed with a view to enhancing detoxification and promoting overall wellbeing. Therefore, the whole diet goal is to regulate the alkaline level of the body using the food we ingest and some herbal supplements. The high alkaline foods are fruits, vegetables, grains, and legumes.

Dr. Sebi recommends that the diet be eaten in three meals a day, with a meal separated by six hours. This ensures that the digestive system is not too overwhelmed and can effectively break down each meal into its parts. The diet also emphasizes the freshness of the food and prefers raw or lightly cooked foods overcooked foods that have been stored for long periods.

He classified food into six categories. These are living foods, raw foods, hybrid foods, dead foods, genetically modified foods, drugs. Living foods are fresh fruits and vegetables. Raw foods are those that are fresh and uncooked, such as raw fruits, greens, etc. Hybrid foods have been steamed or lightly cooked, which preserves most of the food's natural enzymes and nutrients, such as juiced fruits and vegetables. Dead foods are those that have been cooked at a high temperature for a long time. This causes the food to lose most of its nutrients.

He only allows raw and live foods to be consumed. He calls them "electric food," as these foods can charge up your body and give you energy.

Dr. Sebi also suggests that using this diet should get most of their exercise from aerobic activities such as walking or jogging. However, people who are not physically active can also use the diet to add some spices to their daily routine. Some people may have a hard time adjusting and changing their eating habits.

According to Dr. Sebi, after three weeks of following this alkaline diet, you should start noticing some health and well-being changes.

WHAT IS ACIDOSIS?

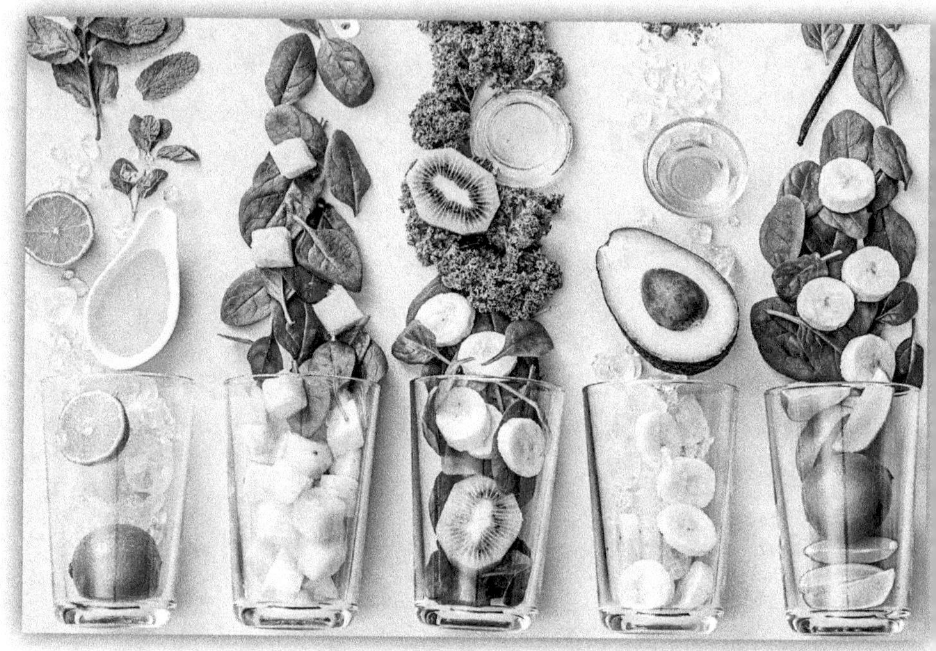

Acidosis

Acidosis occurs when the balance between acid and alkali changes drastically and carries on consistently over time, meaning that too many hydrogen ions are produced. The pH is the value that expresses the degree of a solution's acidity. In our body, it shows us the concentration of hydrogen ions in body fluids. When this state of acid-base balance modifies, even slightly, there are alterations in the normal cellular biochemical and enzymatic reactions that are the basis of life. When too many acid radicals accumulate in the body, a sort of "pollution" occurs, causing disease. And the pH levels run between 0-7.

Types of Acidosis

To find out what kind of acidosis we are facing, this is easily revealed by the targeted organ, and thus by the "defective" organ.

That said the two types of acidosis are:

1. **Respiratory acidosis**. Occurs when there is a build-up of unremoved carbon dioxide in the lungs. Most times, it happens because your lungs are not in their best health due to lung infections or other body and lungs-deteriorating diseases. Examples of conditions that can cause respiratory acidosis are Extreme pneumonia, Asthma, etc.

   Apart from lung diseases, you may be diagnosed with respiratory acidosis when you continuously take drugs that induce sleep. In addition, any cognitive-deteriorating illness that leads to lung issues can be the cause of respiratory acidosis.

   Some many signs and symptoms may appear when you have respiratory acidosis; however, the most common ones include:

   → Chronic headache

   → Tiredness

   → Excessive sleep

   At first, respiratory acidosis might not cause pain. However, if it is neglected, it will become hazardous and may cause the affected person to go into a coma.

2. **Metabolic acidosis**: This is caused by high acidity in the body, which is because of the kidney's inability to release the required

acid or base. The most common causes of metabolic acidosis are:

> Continuous alcohol consumption
> Diseases such as cancer and diabetes
> Insufficient bicarbonate in the body, which promotes extreme vomiting
> The kidney's inability to excrete acids

In addition, metabolic acidosis can result from the continuous intake of medications, such as aspirin, etc.

The most common symptoms of this acidosis are fatigue, frequent vomits, etc.

Metabolic acidosis, if neglected, can cause its victim to go into a coma.

The Negative Effects of High Acidity in Your Body

It's normal that whenever a person says "acid," it will cause bad images to sweep over anyone. This is because the fear and knowledge of the danger of acid are well imprinted in our DNA and evoke the impelling need to run far away from it.

However, acids are impossible to stay away from because they are practically in our bodies. Daily, the production of acids in the body is non-stop. This is because our body gets supplies of acids from our meals, when we take too many short breaths, from our daily exercise sessions, etc. However, you should know that acids in the body are majorly gotten from our diets, and when there is a build-up of these acids in the body, it is detrimental to our well-being. It might leave us quickly stressed, caused by inflammatory diseases like arthritis, skin problems, bowel diseases etc.

You should know high acidity is detrimental to bone durability and strength, muscle growth, tissue formation, joints, and numerous vital body organs.

High acidity leaves the body excessively stressed because the body goes an extra mile to regulate its pH levels; various vital organs work excessively in buffering acidity. When this is insufficient in buffering the body's high acids, the body takes nutrients such as calcium, mostly found in bones, to reduce acidity, making the bones weak and promoting osteoporosis and fractures.

Other effects of high acidity include:

- Terrible breath
- Indigestion
- It causes pain in joints and muscles
- It promotes some skin infections
- It causes chronic migraine
- It encourages cramps
- It promotes various infections caused by fungi

Acidic or Basic?

When we discuss pH levels, we usually think about a diet. However, the issue of acidity is much more complicated than that.

To a large degree, life on earth depends on appropriate pH levels in and around living organisms and cells. For human life to exist, i.e., continue, it requires strictly controlled pH levels of about 7.4.

When we analyze global records over the past 100 years, we see how industrialization has affected the ocean's pH; it dropped because of increasing Carbon dioxide (CO2) deposits. This has had a very retrogressive effect on marine life and may cause the fall of the coral reefs.

On the other hand, the soil's pH in which we grow plants we use for food affects the food's mineral content grown in such soil. The ideal pH of the soil is between 6 and 7. Acidic soil (below 6) has reduced calcium and magnesium, while soil above seven pH may have too much iron, manganese, copper, and zinc. This is why manure and chemical fertilizers are added to soils to increase or neutralize pH levels.

In regards to the human diet, it has undergone a tremendous change over the last few thousand years. Starting with the agricultural revolution more than 10,000 years ago and intensifying since the industrial revolution 200 years ago, there's been a significant drop in potassium (K) and an increase in sodium (Na) and chloride in our diet.

Nutritionists are aware that today's modern diet is deficient in potassium, magnesium, and fiber but rich in simple sugars, saturated fat, and sodium. Compared to what our diet used to be like and how we were genetically programmed to eat, the so-called Western diet is very unhealthy.

The modern diet is particularly unhealthy for middle-aged and senior people because it contributes to a gradual deterioration of kidneys and diet-induced metabolic acidosis. Simply put, this means that although a low-carb, high-protein diet does not affect your blood pH levels; it does affect your urine pH levels and creates ideal conditions for the development of kidney stones.

Health Benefits of Alkaline Diet

The proponents of alkaline diets and scholars supporting high pH balance have argued that high pH is best for the body. You should know that these arguments have been supported by numerous studies, which posit that when the body has a high power of hydrogen (pH) balance, it comes with various health benefits. Some of these benefits are reflected:

On cancer

A study on Alkaline's effect on cancer by a medical practitioner named Tanis Fenton found that high pH levels could improve some cancer drugs' performance.

Sadly, there have been no studies on this subject. However, alkaline diets contain numerous nutrients that prevent cancer; examples of nutrients, such as vitamin A and vitamin C, are known as cancer risk-reducers.

On acid reflux

This disease is caused when acids from the stomach go back towards the food duct.

You should know that when this action happens over an extended period, it could lead to severe health issues such as GERD (gastroesophageal reflux disease).

When the body has a high pH balance, it will help detoxify this acid and reduce gastroesophageal reflux chances.

However, you should know that scholars and dieticians have argued that the stomach's high acidic contents have more usefulness to the body because it allows the natural breakdown of foods and works perfectly in destroying bacteria.

On high blood pressure and diabetes

Studies have shown that a high pH balance reduces excessive blood pressure and works excellently against diabetes.

They argue that making the body more alkaline than acidic rids the blood of viscosity.

Notably, researchers in China have majorly studied the effect of high pH, making it difficult to accept by the world populace because adequate research hasn't been done on the subject matter.

On bones

A good number of studies have been done on the impact of high pH balance on bones.

One major study found that a high pH balance reduces the chances of osteoporosis and bone weakness. Other studies showed that a body with a high pH balance is rich in nutrients like calcium, ensuring bones' durability and strength.

Hence, a high pH balance ensures that individuals have strong and reliable bones, even as they get older.

ALKALINE BLOOD AND THE ROLE OF PH

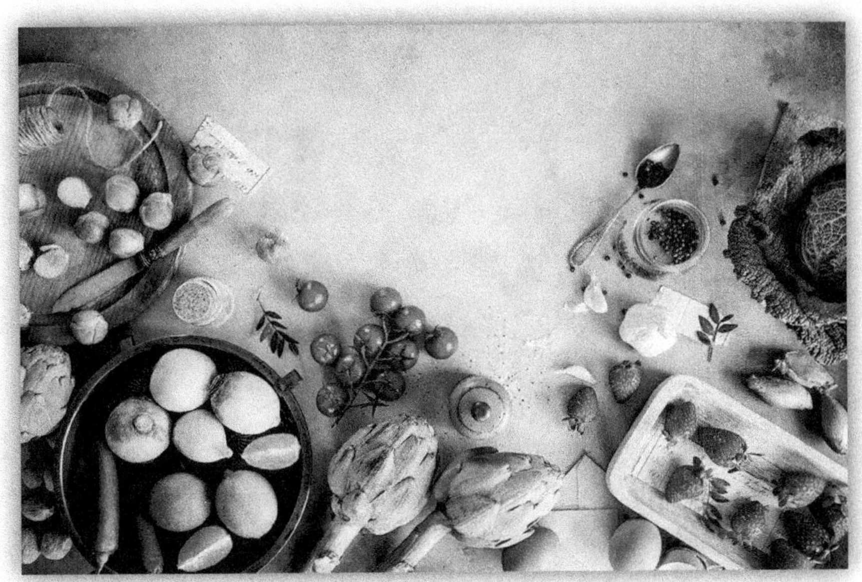

Dr. Sebi's African Bio-Mineral Balance methodology introduced the concept that an acidic body supports disease proliferation, and an alkaline body protects against disease. The issue is a bit more complex, which gave people who wanted to be divisive ammunition to attack his methodology. More specifically, acidic blood supports the proliferation of disease. Science supports that there are alkaline parts of the body and acidic parts.

- **The Stomach:** Has a pH of 1.35-3.5, but the "Mucous Neck Cells" that are right below the stomach's surface have a neutral pH.

- **Skin:** The outer layer has a pH of around 4 to protect it from the bacteria in the environment, and the inner layer has a pH of around 6.9.

- **Vagina:** Has a pH of around 4.5 to protect against microbial overgrowth.

- **Pancreas:** PH is between 8 – 8.3.

- **Intestines:** Small intestine has a range of 6-7.4pH, and the large intestine has a pH range of 5.7-6.7.

- Blood: Has a pH range between 7.35 and 7.45 (7.4 is the number commonly used).

Alkaline and acid are opposite sides of the pH scale. The scale for pH ranges from 0pH to 14pH. 0pH represents the highest acidic level, and 14pH represents the highest alkaline level. 7.0pH is neutral. Though different body areas are acidic, it is essential to eat alkaline foods to maintain a blood pH of around 7.4. The blood's pH is the reference point for the homeostasis or optimal functioning of the body's organs.

The body works diligently to keep the blood in a slightly alkaline state near a pH of 7.4 to support homeostasis and health. pH stands for "potential hydrogen" and is the ability of molecules to attract hydrogen ions. Too many hydrogen ions floating around the bloodstream make the blood acidic and interfere with the body's proper oxygenation. Eating meat, dairy, processed foods, and even highly hybridized starchy plant foods acidify the blood because of their molecule structure. They also lack vital minerals, vitamins, and phytonutrients the body needs to perform metabolic functions properly.

The body uses oxygen to release energy from nutrients so cells can use components from the nutrients to heal, repair, and sustain themselves. Without the required energy, organ function is compromised, resulting in sluggishness and illness. An acidic environment wreaks havoc on the immune system's white blood cells and causes them to go into a dormant state. This allows bacteria, viruses, and fungi to increase, attack weakened organs, and interfere with normal and healthy bodily functions.

The blood's pH reflects the health of the whole body. Suppose the body doesn't get enough alkaline material to maintain a blood pH of around 7.4. In that case, the body will leach alkaline material from other body areas to maintain homeostasis. As an example, the body will leach calcium from bones to maintain the blood's proper pH at the bones' expense. This leaching can lead to osteoporosis development and result in a reduction of bone density and bone fractures.

The body uses buffering mechanisms, like the kidney's bicarbonate production, to maintain the blood's needed alkalinity. When those systems are overwhelmed, the body finds its way, leaching alkaline material from fluids and tissues throughout the body. The leaching includes other areas in the body, leaving them susceptible to pathogens and toxins. The body will compromise other body areas because it is vitally important to maintain a blood pH of around 7.4. Metabolic acidosis, which happens when the blood's pH drops under 7.4, is highly to avoid as it is dangerous. The chronic consumption of acidic foods risks the entire body's health and supports disease manifestation in cells and mitochondria.

Natural plant foods properly alkalize the blood, maintain its desired pH, and support an inhospitable environment to disease. Eating natural plant foods optimally helps homeostasis or peak the operation of organs. The plant's source of nutrients is minerals they absorb from the earth, water, and air. Each type of plant comprises different combinations and ratios of nutrients, which is determined by its genetic structure.

Nourishing oneself in a varied and natural way, preferring pure nutritional sources, promotes the oxygenation of the body and brings vital lymph. What happens in plants happens to us, we are part of this living Microcosm and we are strongly connected to it.

Macronutrients of plant foods

Plant foods are full of micronutrients: minerals, phytonutrients, vitamins, and the carbohydrate macronutrient. To support cell health and energy the body uses these primary nutrients. The chemical structure of protein and animal fat also differs from plant fat and protein that alkalizes the blood instead of acidifying it.

Plants' minerals and vitamins help them to grow strong and vibrant, while plants' phytonutrients protect them against environmental pathogens. Plants absorb the sun's energy through photosynthesis, convert its energy into physical forms of energy it uses for growth, and support chemical processes.

People consume the plants and absorb their natural balance of elements, compounds, and energy manifested in their minerals, vitamins, phytonutrients, carbohydrates, fats, and proteins. As with plants, the human body is derived from these same elements and compounds. When people consume plant life, they consume elements and compounds that support the healthy function of organs. Natural plants' chemical structure has a chemical affinity with the body, so their digestion doesn't produce harmful.

Meat, dairy, and processed foods are deficient in microminerals, many vitamins, and phytonutrients necessary to support optimal organ function. The food industry was aware of the deficiency and developed vitamin and mineral supplements. Plant foods naturally provide nutrients in combinations the body recognizes, but artificial supplementation does not. Numerous studies have shown that the nutrients in plant-based foods supports health.

A well-balanced, whole-food, alkaline plant-based diet is naturally high in minerals, vitamins, and phytonutrients. The diet is also high in natural carbohydrates. The body burns quickly for energy. Natural carbohydrates are the body's primary fuel source. The diet is also naturally low in fat and protein and provides a ratio of 70% carbohydrates, 10% fat, and 20% protein. This is the ratio nature provides to support the healthy function of organs optimally.

An alkaline plant-based diet supplies the small amount of fat needed to support bodily functions, such as providing insulation for organs, storage of fat-soluble vitamins, and supporting brain function, growth, and cell functions. It also supplies the small amount of protein needed to support antibody and enzyme production, transport of components, building and maintaining cells, and transmitting messages throughout the body. An alkaline plant-based diet provides fully supported the longstanding recommended daily allowance (RDA) of 10% protein, on a plant-basis. This was the recommendation for protein up until industry pressure influenced the Food and Nutrition Board to change the recommendation in 2002.

WHAT IS THE MUCUS. WHY IS IT RESPONSIBLE FOR MAJOR DISEASES?

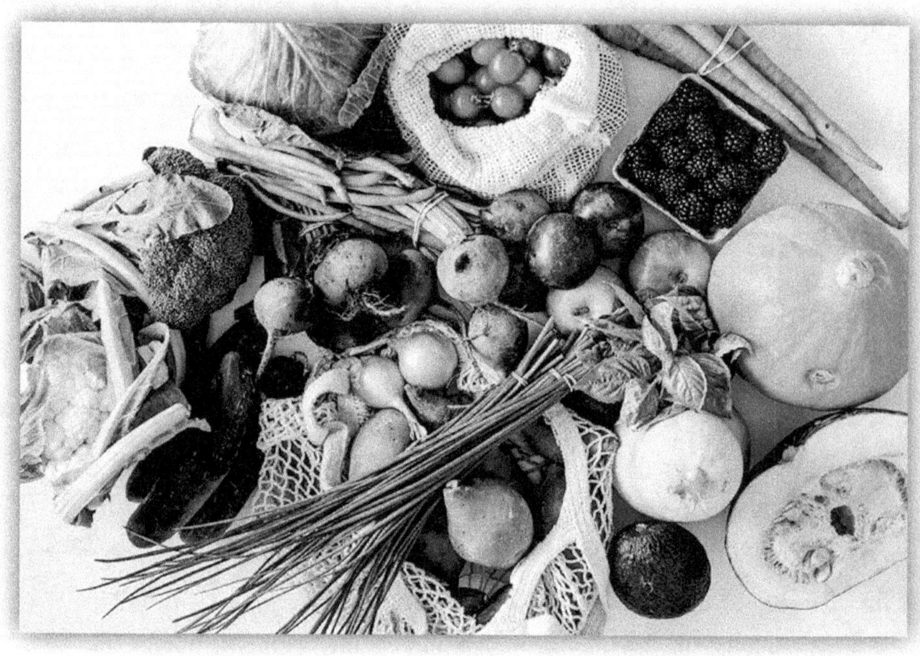

The creation of mucus is an essential aspect of our bodies. Each day, the body constantly produces doses of mucus for a wide range of functions. Typically, this production is for the benefit of the body. Unfortunately, as with everything in life, it can become negative when the production becomes excessive.

This idea is one that underpins Dr. Sebi's road to a healthy diet. Unfortunately, there has been a misconstruction of the role of mucus within the body. Even worse, it continues to receive limited attention when it is, in fact, a core component of healthy living. Precisely, where the mucus membrane is allowed to function properly, it performs a wide range of functions that keep the body in the best condition possible.

On the other hand, where it is pressured due to a wide variety of activities, including poor diet, it results in excessive mucus production, making the body susceptible to illness. It is necessary that you understand the role of mucus in the body and the various dietary options that can compromise the mucus membrane.

What is Mucus?

This refers to a stringy and slippery fluid substance that various lining tissues within the body produce. While this is sometimes perceived as unwanted, the reality is that mucus is actually essential to normal body functioning. This is because it performs a wide range of essential functions within the main organs.

Mucus has various components, with the most prominent being mucin. This mucin works as a selective barrier, viscous material, or lubricant. In this case, the function it performs will depend on the mucin's structure.

Note that the body produces a significant amount of mucus. For instance, each day, it is estimated that the body produces a minimum of 1 liter. This can then rise to as much as 1.5 liters in some cases. However, the good news is that we hardly notice the production of this mucus. As we stated, they perform essential functions within the body that makes this significant production desirable, but the body does it silently...in most cases.

The mucus gland is responsible for the production of mucus. It is located in various body sites and includes the lungs, sinuses, throat, nose, cervix, gastrointestinal tract, and mouth.

The Problem with Mucus

So far, it has become more evident that mucus is not just a disgusting element that should not be in your body. It is a vital component constantly produces by the body to keep it in shape.

So, where does the problem come from, and how does this important body component become an issue?

As we have illustrated so far, the body needs a constant balance of all its constituents to function effectively. Too little of an important component, and you will have a problem. On the other hand, too much of anything, and there is still a problem.

There is a need to find a balance between alkaline and acidic intake. Well, this is also the case with mucus within the body.

While mucus performs a wide range of positive functions within the body, the problem arises when mucus production exceeds the natural level. As Dr. Sebi would rightly say, this causes a wide range of problems within the body. For instance, too much mucus within the joints becomes a problem. While the mucus should ordinarily hydrate the joint, it begins to cause issues, which we now know as arthritis.

Excessive mucus production becomes an issue as it brings discomfort in the various areas where it occurs. For instance, it can cause a runny nose, sore throat, cough, sinus headache, sore throat, and nasal congestion.

Still, it can cause various intestinal problems and change the structure of the probiotic bacterial composition. Western medicine would have you believe that excessive mucus rarely translates to a serious medical problem. However, as Dr. Sebi has established through his teachings, excessive mucus is, in fact, the cause of all diseases.

The presence of excessive mucus in the bronchial is what causes what we now know as bronchitis. If you are experiencing eye issues, then the brain is seeing more mucus production than it is healthy for it. So, it becomes evident that excessive production of mucus within the body is not just another issue. In fact, a serious issue deserves your attention.

Factors Responsible for Excessive Mucus Production

- **Respiratory Infection** — our body is not always immune to infections. In turn, this infection can contribute to excessive mucus production, which makes us more vulnerable to other infections.

- **Allergic Reactions** — allergic reactions push your body outside of its natural state. In turn, this can lead the body to react through the increased production of mucus.

- **Toxins And Pollutants** - it involves a wide range of environmental factors that pollute the body system — for instance, living in an environment that sees an increased production of carbon monoxide and other pollutants like smoke will surely increase mucus production.

- **Dietary Practices** — Various food substances and beverages can cause your body to start producing mucus at an alarming rate.

Dr. Sebi's Detoxifying and Cleansing Diets to Remove Infected Mucus

Dr. Sebi did not identify or recommend pharmaceuticals for the condition. He appeared to be a culinary expert and made nutrition-related proposals. At least one hour before starting your medicine, it is advised that you take the products so that the nutrients given will be completely assimilated.

Products from Dr. Sebi are labeled as food for natural vegetation cells. Therefore, nourishing the cells will also reduce the sense of hunger, in fact it is recommended to take the herbs at least an hour before eating.

The anti-inflammatory pathway doesn't just deal with the symptoms; it aims to investigate the origins of the disease. And the origin of the disease is mucus, that defensive weapon that the body deploys when it needs to keep high inflammatory levels under control and incorporate large numbers of toxins. The disease will occur in the body where the mucus has accumulated. Because natural food compounds are designed to remove mucus from a specific part of the body, it is often important to get them working in synergy, cleaning the body on the whole. The special and exclusive features of the compounds of Dr. Sebi are the way they function to cleanse and nourish the whole body.

You will successfully reverse pathologies through this method. As the herbs used have a natural origin, the substances begin to unleash their cleansing properties 14 days after they are first taken. Adhering to the dietary recommendations is an equally significant part of Dr. Sebi's diet policy. In combination with dietary improvements, Dr. Sebi's herbal compounds function to give the body the right climate to maintain optimum wellness. It also aims to achieve the most positive effects on your well-being by consuming a gallon of natural spring water every day.

PRINCIPLES OF ALKALINE FOOD

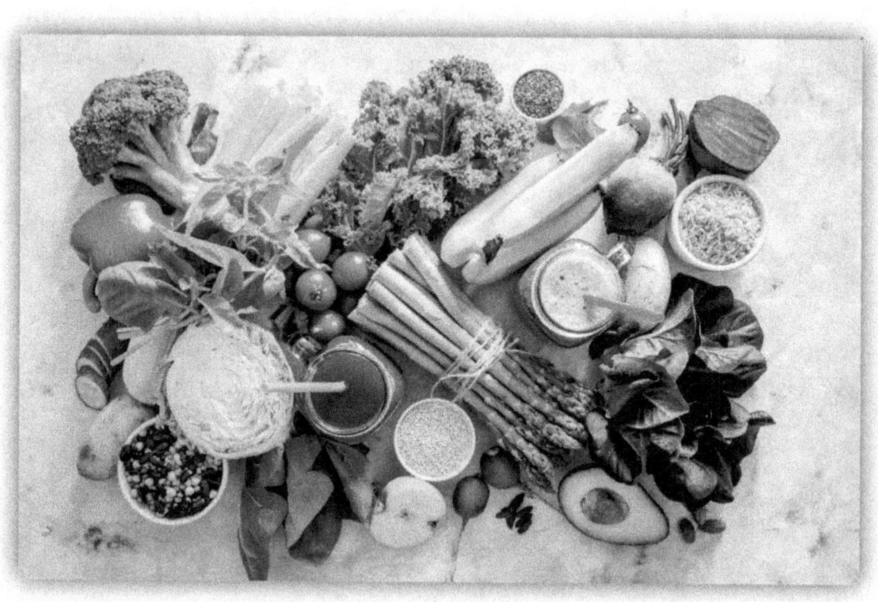

The alkaline diet, otherwise called Alkaline Acid Diet, is diet-dependent on the utilization of nourishment. For example, natural products, vegetables, roots, nuts, and vegetables, however, maintain a strategic distance from dairy, meat, grains, and salts. As of late, this diet has picked up fame among diet and nourishment experts and creators. It is still in banter on the productivity of the alkaline diet because there is no solid proof that the alkaline diet can decrease certain diseases.

Organic products, vegetables, roots, nuts, and vegetables are a piece of an alkaline diet. This is because this nourishment discharged alkaline in the wake of being processed, assimilated, and used. Then again, dairy, meat, grains, and salts produce acid after the procedures. Nourishment is classified as acid-delivering or alkaline-creating dependent on their pH (intensity of Hydrogen) values, where pH 0 - 6 is acidic, pH 8 - 14 is alkaline, and pH 7 is nonpartisan (water). Consequently, the alkaline diet alludes to the menu of having a more significant amount of alkaline-delivering nourishment.

Our blood has a pH somewhere in the range of 7.35 and 7.45, which is marginally alkaline. The alkaline diet depends on the pH level of our blood, and any food that is high in acid-delivering nourishment will disorganize the equalization. This means, if we introduce acidifying foods, at the time when the body is trying to rebalance the pH harmony in the blood, the acidity of the food will cause the loss of crucial minerals, such as potassium, magnesium, calcium, and sodium. The irregularity may make us more vulnerable and susceptible to various up & downs due to pH imbalance. By consuming purely alkaline foods, this does not happen, the blood values remain in balance, and the body is free to continue doing its normal work.

What Are the Strict Rules to Follow?

You should know that this program is entirely plant-based, a vegan diet. It consists of nuts and seeds, grains, fruits, vegetables, herbs, and oils. Consuming animal products is wholly prohibited. The rules surrounding this diet are stringent. They hinge on keeping individuals away from processed foods and animal products while encouraging them to take the listed supplements. These rules are not scientifically grounded nutritional guidelines.

There are eight rules to follow:

1. You are only allowed to eat the foods listed in the nutritional guide.

2. You are supposed to drink 2 liters of water every day.

3. Doctor Sebi's supplements are to be consumed an hour before taking any medication.

4. Animal products (including meat, milk, eggs, etc.) are not allowed.

5. Alcohol consumption is not permitted.

6. Do not consume wheat products at all. You are only supposed to eat "natural growing grains" that are outlined in the nutritional guide.

7. The use of microwaves is not permitted, as it is considered to kill the nutrients present in foods.

8. Canned and seedless fruits are prohibited.

Benefits of Dr. Sebi Diet for All the Diseases

➤ **Give Protection to Bone Density and Muscle Mass**

Taking minerals into your body system plays a significant role in maintaining and developing your body's bones. Research has proved to the truth that the more alkaline-rich fruits and vegetables you take regularly, the better you get protected from experiencing reduced bone muscle and strength, known as Sarcopenia. An alkaline diet does when you take to help balance the ratios of the various minerals in the body necessary for bone building and the maintenance of a lean muscle mass.

The minerals that an alkaline diet balances are Phosphate, Magnesium, and Calcium. Another benefit of an alkaline diet is the improvement in the production of vitamin D absorption and growth hormones, which help, in further protecting the bones and fighting against many chronic diseases.

➢ **Reduce the Risk of Hypertension and Stroke**

Another great benefit of eating an alkaline diet is reducing the risk of stroke and hypertension that an individual is prone to have. A typical alkaline diet has an anti-aging effect. A robust result of the anti-aging effects is that it drastically reduces inflammation and fosters hormone production growth. This has been verified to help improve cardiovascular health and give the body defense against typical health challenges like hypertension, high cholesterol, stroke, kidney stones, and possible memory loss.

➢ **Reduce Chronic Pain and Inflammation**

There is a correlation between alkaline diets and a drastic reduction in levels of chronic pain. Chronic acidosis is dangerous to the human health system. It is the primary cause of headaches, chronic back pain, joint pain, inflammation, menstrual symptoms, and muscle spasms.

Cases abound that show the health benefits of alkaline diets suffering from chronic pains. A study conducted showed a significant level of decrease in the pain experienced by patients suffering from chronic back pain when they were supplements containing alkaline daily for four weeks.

➢ **Weight Loss**

This diet was not made with weight loss in mind, but you will see weight loss because it is extremely restrictive. One of the main reasons that this diet is effective in reducing weight is that it makes people stop consuming Western foods, which are highly caloric, oily, and sugary.

Weight loss occurs when you eat less or equal amounts of calories that you can burn. If you follow this diet, which is low in sugar, fat, and processed foods, you can get your perfect body.

➢ **Improves Kidney Function**

Acidic diets mostly affect the health of the kidneys and damages the layers inside the organ system. To promote kidney health, the pH of the urine must not be acidic.

By consuming a lot of alkaline food, and removing acidic foods from our daily routine, we can reach the pH at which our kidneys remain safe and healthy. Alkaline diets do not affect the pH of the blood, but they can significantly affect the urine. Drinking a lot of water alongside this diet can improve kidneys even more. It's important to mention that, if you suffer from any chronic kidney disease, then this diet is not suitable, and you should always first consult a doctor. Who can indicate whether it is appropriate to undertake an alkaline diet.

> **Reduces the Risk of Cancer**

There are no significant studies to show that an alkaline diet leads to decreased cases of cancer.

However, studies show that if a person were to eat less meat, and increase their consumption of fresh fruits and vegetables, then that person is at a lower risk of cancer. Another study also showed that having more vitamins, like vitamin C, in your diet could prevent cancer. Generally, eating more fruits and vegetables and consuming less high fatty and sugary foods, leads to a reduction in developing acidosis-related diseases, whose most potent expression is cancer.

> **Reduces the Risk of Heart Disease**

Heart disease is the major cause of death in the world. It is mainly caused by eating many fats and oily foods, which results in the development of plaque and blockage of arteries. In this diet, the consumption of fats decreases significantly, decreasing the chances of developing heart disease.

It has also been shown that growth hormones are related to decreased rates of heart disease. An alkaline diet increases the levels of growth hormones, so, in turn; it decreases heart disease as well.

> **Reduces the Risk of Muscle Degradation**

When we grow old or stop using our muscles, we tend to increase muscle loss. However, a study conducted in 2013 showed that people who follow an alkaline diet could decrease muscle degradation.

> **Increases Intestinal Health**

You can eat on this diet whole grain and a list of nuts and seeds. It contributes to an increase in fiber intake, which increases the health of small and large intestines. It helps manage regular bowel movements, which reduces the risk of developing many diseases.

> **Decreases the Harmful Effects of Processed Foods**

Processed foods have been linked to increased sugar intake and fat content. They also contain many calories but have very low nutritional value. Many additives and preservatives that have no purpose in our bodies are eliminated from our diets if we strictly avoid processed foods. The alkaline diet helps reduce the effects of industrial foods and get rid of the toxic load much faster.

> **It Helps the Brain**

The growth hormone is related to a better heart condition and helps manage the health of the mind. It is related to an increase in memory and cognition. Eating a healthy diet rich in fruits, and vegetables leads to better brain functioning.

> **It May Improve Back Pain**

Alkaline minerals are related to reducing back pain, but whether alkaline foods provide the same results has yet to be determined. There is a decent chance that the diet has similar effects.

> **Decreases the Level of Inflammation**

Diets rich in fresh fruits and vegetables promote a decrease in oxidative stress and inflammation. This leads to less discomfort and fewer diseases developing in our bodies.

Counteracting inflammation is one of the main purposes of this diet, as high levels of inflammation mean disease development in every system and organ.

> **Prevent Deficiency in Magnesium and Increases Vitamin Absorption**

Magnesium plays an essential role in the human body, as an increase in its quantity is necessary for the proper functioning of all the human body's enzymes, and processes. Deficiency in magnesium content will result in headaches, anxiety, heart complications, muscle pains, and sleep troubles. Magnesium is also needed by the body to activate vitamin D and prevent Vitamin D deficiency, necessary for the functioning of the endocrine and overall body immunity.

> **Improving Cancer Protection and Immune Function**

The body needs minerals in disposing of waste or in oxygenating the body. However, when there is a shortage of the required minerals in the cells, the body suffers. Vitamin absorption is zeroed off whenever there is a mineral loss in the body. In addition, toxins and pathogens will pile up in the body, thereby weakening the immune system. However, with alkaline diets, that cannot happen as research has proved that cancerous cells' death happens more in an alkaline body.

Alkaline diets will help in decreasing inflammation and the possible risks associated with dangerous diseases such as cancer.

- **Help You in Maintaining a Healthy Balanced Weight**

To limit the acidic content in your body and protect your body from the risks associated with obesity you can eat more diets that are alkaline.

This is possible as alkaline diets decrease the levels of Leptin, and inflammation, which has a direct effect on your hunger, and fat-burning capacities.

How Much Weight You Lose

These days, you come across so many weight-loss diets and gyms on every street, but people all over the world are becoming overweight despite this, and this is being considered an epidemic. We all think that the usual cause of obesity is consuming more than the amount of food our body needs, but this is also a good point to consider: eating a lot might not necessarily be the cause of someone's obesity since some people eat a lot but never put on weight. However, eating a large amount of the wrong types of acidifying foods will definitely result in weight gain.

The Dr. Sebi alkaline diet helps your body to function at an optimum level in order to help you lose weight naturally, and the good news about it is that it doesn't involve cutting out foods or counting calories, which are the common reasons why many diets are unsustainable in the long-term. We often look for quick fixes that don't last. For example, the yo-yo diet, where you might lose weight for a few weeks, then regains it immediately you stop the diet. The Dr. Sebi alkaline diet aims to change how we think about food and our eating habits for the long-term, possibly for life.

One thing never forget is that exercising is always another focal step in your weight loss journey. Keep exercising, keep running or biking or going to the gym, or whatever, together with the alkaline diet, will generally help our body to rid itself of excess weight naturally. The first step to take before deciding what changes to make to our diet to improve health is to know our pH level and keep it monitored over time as we move and eat alkaline and naturally.

ASPECTS TO CONSIDER ABOUT DR. SEBI'S DIET

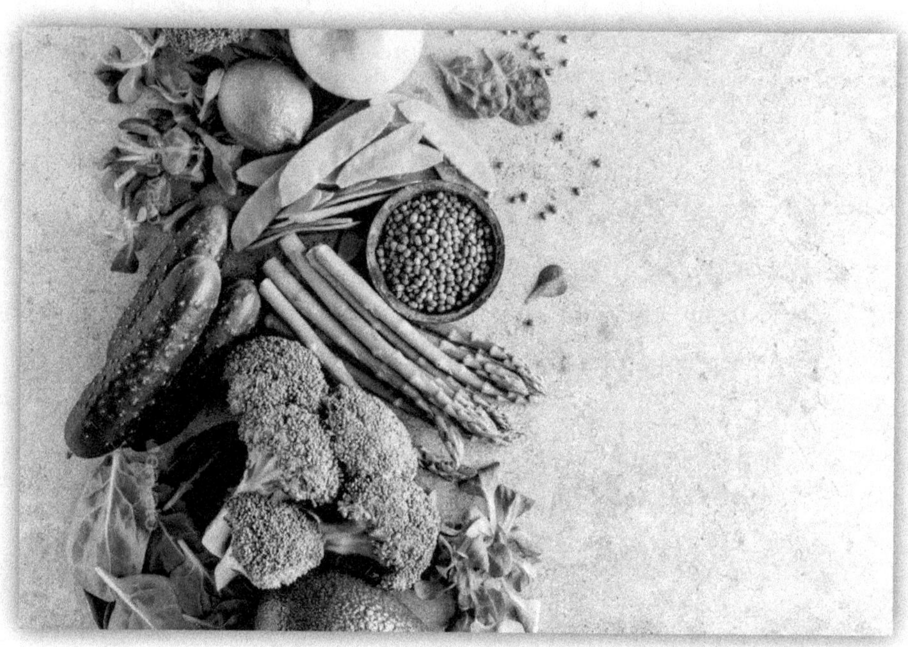

Dr. Sebi's Pure Diet is quite restrictive, as it is a deep detox that is supposed to cleanse your body, flush it of inflammation and return it to its healthy alkaline state. Which in a short time is no problem at all. However, if you are planning to follow it for a long period, you should consider that there might be some deficiencies that you need to pay attention to.

Avoid VIT B12 deficiencies

Vitamin B-12 is an essential nutrient for the health of the nerves and blood cells and the development of DNA.

In general, people who have vegan or vegetarian diets and older adults are at risk of B-12 deficiency. Doctors generally consider taking B-12 supplements for people who do not eat animal products.

Symptoms of B-12 deficiency include tiredness, exhaustion, and tingling in the hands and feet. There is also a chance of pernicious anemia, which prevents the body from producing sufficiently healthy red blood cells. It is recommended to take VIT B12 supplements to compensate for a possible deficiency.

Low Protein

Dr. Sebi did not endorse the word or definition of protein because it clashed with his approach to Healing. Instead, he concentrated on minerals or elements. Elements like nitrogen are the building blocks of muscles and enzymes. Nitrogen-based systems in the body, such as muscles and enzymes, are supported by the assimilation of nitrogen compounds. People have been compelled to think they need to get these nitrogen compounds by eating meat, and this is not true. Plants contain nitrogen-based compounds such as meat, which are referred to as proteins. These nitrogenous organic compounds consist of massive amino acid molecules that are components of muscle, hair, collagen, enzymes, and antibodies.

Protein helps improve the wellbeing of the brain, muscles, bones, hormones, and DNA in the diet.

Protein helps improve brain, muscle, bone, hormone and DNA wellness in the diet.

According to existing guidelines, females over 19 years of age are expected to have a daily protein intake of 46 grams (g), whereas males of the same age are expected to eat 56 g.

Some foods included in Dr. Sebi's diet contain protein. For example, 100 g of hemp seed contains 31.56 g of protein, while the same amount of walnut contains 16.67 g of protein. If we compare, 100 g of oven-roasted chicken breast contains 16.79 g of nutrients.

Research indicates that it is necessary to eat a wide variety of plant foods to absorb enough amino acids that are primary components of protein. This may be difficult when you follow Dr. Sebi's diet.

Without a doubt, this alkaline diet is lacking in proteins. But we must not forget that this type of diet is the most suitable in a detox path, necessary to deeply cleanse the body from all dangerous and inflammatory waste and toxins, which have favored the origin and development of a disease. Only this type of diet, away from the consumption of animal foods allows a complete regeneration of the body.

And this does not necessarily presuppose to be followed for a long period, but for what is necessary to the function of promoting a state of health. This can also be a detoxification of the organs at each change of season, or after an illness and medication intake, or a detox period of several weeks to return to the desired form and shape.

The Dr Sebi Diet does not allow animal proteins, eggs, dairy products or even soy. It also excludes most beans and legumes. The only products that include some protein in the diet are some "natural grains", hemp seeds, walnuts, and Brazil nuts.

Protein is a significant component of every cell in the body, and the body uses protein to help build and regenerate tissue. They are an essential building block of bone, muscle, skin, blood and cartilage. Limiting major food groups and macronutrients, over a long period, can contribute to nutritional deficiencies and malnutrition.

The use of fruits and vegetables is promoted, although possibilities are quite limited.

Dr Sebi focuses primarily on his supplements, which make tall claims that they can " promote the healing process" and "revitalize and help grow intracellular connections." This makes it more interesting to know what you get from her proprietary blends and to find out what exactly is in her supplements.

Compensate for Deficiency of Omega 3 Fatty Acids

Omega-3 fatty acids are the main components of the cell membrane. They are supporting:

- The health of the brain, heart, and eye
- Energy: Energy
- The Immunity System

Dr. Sebi's diet includes plant sources of omega-3s, such as hemp seeds and walnuts.

However, the body from animal sources more readily absorbs these acids. A 2019 study shows that the vegan diet contains little or no two omega-3 fatty acids unless a person takes a supplement.

Anyone who follows Dr. Sebi's diet may benefit from taking an omega-3 supplement.

HOW TO PURIFY THE LIVER, GUT, AND INTESTINE

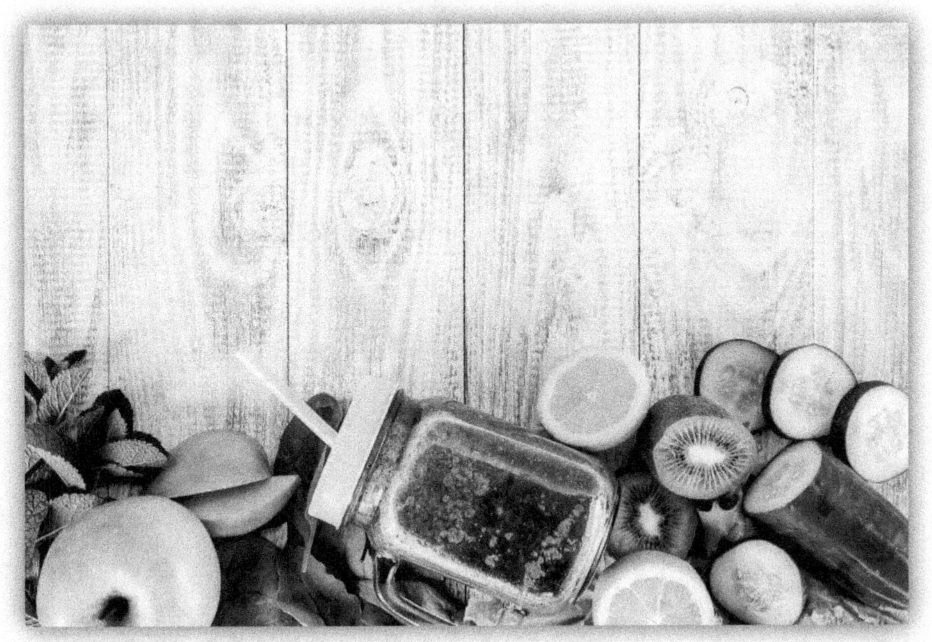

Detoxing the Liver

Human anatomy has been designed to lead a balanced life in an exceptional way, but owing to our chaotic, sometimes out-of-control "modern world lifestyle," and its environment, our bodies, and minds are subject to a constant influx of toxins. Our body functions are at considerable risk under this strain because they are sometimes weakened and may quickly cede to diseases and illnesses. A detox is like pressing a reset button on the body. This gives a break to our bodies and brains and slows down the digestive tract. Our bodies go into recovery mode after detox so that we can concentrate on self-care and healing.

Importance of Liver

The liver is the largest organ of the body at about 1.4 kg and conducts a variety of important functions, including:

- Helps produce vitamin D required to produce hormones

- Removes toxic chemicals, microbes, and unwanted hormones from the body

- Stores vitamins and minerals that include iron and vitamin B12 as well.

- Processes the fats, proteins, and carbohydrates from the food you consume so you can get the energy and nutrients from whatever you consume.

- Creates products that are used by your immune system to protect your body from infections.

- Stores the sugar (glycogen) for future use when energy is required by your body.

- Thus, you can see, your liver, and your hormonal well-being, is incredibly essential to your overall health. If it doesn't perform well, you need to take the measures to help detoxify your liver and regain its healthy function. What you consume, drink, but even breathe and come in touch with through your skin, and it then reaches your bloodstream, the body needs to process it. Therefore, maintaining a balanced lifestyle and adopting a healthy diet is incredibly essential to your well-being, especially your liver's health and well-being.

-

Method to Cleanse Your Liver

Eat a High Fiber Diet

It's no surprise that fiber plays a crucial role in maintaining a healthy weight. Fiber also plays a significant role in keeping a healthy liver, though. The liver helps produce bile. In the large intestines, fiber binds to bile. Bile carries the fat-soluble toxins stored away from the liver so they can be removed during bowel movements. Leafy greens like kale, spinach, and broccoli are filled with fiber. In addition, don't forget about your delicious fruit. However, make sure both of your fruits and veggies are organic for better results.

Go on a Diet of Juice

When you consume heavily refined foods full of sugar, carbohydrates, and chemicals, the liver has to work very hard to do its job. That's why it's essential to give your liver 2–3 days' rest. Going on a juice quickly and consuming fruit, vegetables, and healthy liquids are the best way to give your liver and digestive system a rest. Not only can you do your liver a favor, but all the nutrients that your body requires to remain balanced will be consumed too.

Wash Your Liver

Liver flushing is one of the most traditional ways of purifying and detoxifying your liver. Liver flushing is an old method that allows you to "flush" out toxins, parasites, gallstones, and by-products from food. Usually, a liver flush involves drinking or eating an eclectic blend of herbs, teas, juices, and oil. It mostly takes 2-3 days to flush your liver to have it again function as usual. It's imperative, though, that you eat a diet full of organic fruits and cruciferous vegetables to keep your liver in good condition.

Fasting

Just as your bowels, need a break, so does your liver. Your liver is always up and running, eliminating toxins and processing the carbohydrates, fats, and proteins you digest. Sometimes it is best to give your liver a break and to go on a juice quickly. When you don't eat for a couple of days, the body immediately begins the removal cycle and removes toxins spontaneously and effortlessly. Moving quickly also allows the liver and other internal organs to regain balance.

Herbs

- Milk thistle — this potent herb, is considered to be packed with antioxidants that protect against damage to your liver. Those antioxidants function by preventing the liver from consuming toxins.
- Dandelion root — this small root serves as a natural diuretic in addition to blood and liver purification.
- Artichoke extract — helps to increase liver bile flow.
- Fenugreek — composed of potent antioxidants that clean the liver naturally.
- Yellow dock — a strong herb purifying blood widely used in every part of the world.
- Licorice root — supports the digestive and liver health systems.

Your liver's job is to filter all the damaging particles out of your body. External factors such as smoking, poor diet, and toxins can, however, damage your liver and hinder its ability to perform its job. That's why detoxifying your organ regularly is essential. Remember this spring to change your oil!

Toxins Effect on the Liver

Now the liver is metabolizing the hormones and other compounds through; what is known as phase 1 and phase 2 pathways, two main stages.

If your blood is very toxic, it can have a detrimental impact on your liver's well-being, and you might be suffering from what's considered a congested liver.

Symptoms with badly clogged liver include:

- Hormonal imbalance

- Weight gain

- Skin issues of rosacea, acne, dermatitis, rashes, psoriasis, and eczema

- Exhaustion

- Impaired digestion

- Chemical sensitivities

In addition, possibly inflammation in the upper right portion of the abdomen where the liver is situated.

Fatty Liver Disease

Furthermore, you will increase your risk of dying from what is considered non-alcoholic fatty liver disease from an unhealthy diet and lifestyle, which is when you get so much fat in your liver. The fatty liver disorder is now America's most prevalent form of dreadful liver disease, affecting 70 million Americans — that's one in three people.

It may contribute to hepatic cancer, liver disease, and death at its worst. The warning factors for fatty liver disease now include:

- Type 2 diabetes and pre-diabetes

- Being overweight

- Possessing elevated amounts of fat in the body, such as cholesterol and triglycerides

- Recovering from other diseases, such as hepatitis C

- Exposure to contaminants

- Metabolic syndrome

- High blood pressure

Research has been conducted on 9,000 American people who have been followed for about 13 years. It showed that there is a close correlation between consumption of cholesterol (from the diet they consume, including, for example, animal products such as eggs and meat) and hospitalization and mortality from liver cancer and cirrhosis. That is how dietary cholesterol can oxidize, creating harmful and carcinogenic consequences. So consuming animal products is another way the liver will sustain damage, and that may lead to liver cirrhosis (liver scarring) and even hepatic cancer.

Cleansing the Intestines

The Role Played By Toxins in Your Digestion Issues

Our lives are jammed full of ever more dangerous chemicals. Our food, domestic cleaners, cosmetics, self-care products, and the air itself have environmental pollutants. Today only low-grade contaminants occur on most typically cultivated vegetables and fruits.

Healthy bodies detoxify all that may be dangerous to eliminate. Yet over time, our bodies inflict harmful effects; subjected to the contaminants. The contaminants in your body will trigger your digestive system to quit functioning properly, resulting in gaining weight and a host of other problems.

What happens if the digestive system doesn't operate properly?

If your digestive tract is not operating well, contaminants overload the liver. Some contaminants can live long, which can make us feel ill and lethargic. The metabolism of the body slows down, and the accumulation of contaminants triggers fluid accumulation, bloating, and puffiness before you realize it.

Symptoms:

- Gas/Burping
- Sore skin
- Leaky intestine
- Heartburn
- Weight increase
- Bloating

- Stomach discomfort
- Persistent swelling
- Constipation
- Nausea
- Appetite loss
- Diarrhea and vomiting
- Extreme fatigue
- Mental distress
- Low-grade diseases
- Puffy or bags around the eyes
- Allergies

How Toxins Lead to Digestive Problems

The more contaminants you encounter in your life, the more detrimental effects body parts face. Your Food and environment decide how high your toxic load is over time, and then the toxicity triggers inflammation, which contributes to gain weight.

How these toxins induce digestive problems is a complex procedure, which mainly happens in your liver, which is responsible for transforming contaminants into extremely reactive metabolites before these contaminants are fully excreted from the body. Although your body's liver is most damaged by toxins — the gallbladder, intestines, and pancreas are all important organs that retain toxins in your digestive system.

A healthy digestive processes break down the diet to absorb the necessary vitamins and minerals that they can expel the unusable products in your everyday bowel movements. If this one-way mechanism will not function well, people more commonly experience:

- Nausea
- Leaky gut
- Indigestion
- Diarrhea
- Irritable bowel syndrome
- Constipation
-
- Allergies, mainly in food
- Hemorrhoids
- Obesity and weight gain
- Dehydration
- Nutrient deficiencies
- Diabetes
- Ulcers
- Small intestinal overgrowth
- Persistent diarrhea
- Signs of liver disease
- Skin issues like Psoriasis or Eczema
- Hemolytic uremic syndrome
- Brain and Heart problems
- Autoimmune conditions, like Multiple Sclerosis, Crohn's Disease, Celiac Disease, Lupus, Rheumatoid Arthritis, and more

How to Treat Issues Related to Digestive Tract Caused by Toxins

The best way to cure digestive issues induced by contaminants is to eliminate or reduce the intake, to clear toxic accumulation from the body.

There are also different methods that you should seek to rid the body of contaminants before they induce stomach problems. Full body detoxification is also an effective remedy for toxin-induced digestive disorders, whereas other alternative approaches such as consuming the correct foods and utilizing supplements to enhance gastrointestinal well-being can help.

Your body, though, can only detoxify adequately with the correct food, lots of sleep, and good hygiene.

Paybacks of Detox for Digestive Issues

A digestive detox uses natural foods to wash away contaminants from the body. Digestive health is important to your well-being, so you can find advantages by cleansing up your body:

- Intestines
- Colon
- Liver

Detoxes can remove the body's toxic substances so pollutants until the pounds pile up. They improve your digestive well-being, too. Any contaminants within you will normally grow removed before they have enough time to inflict damage.

A detox cleanse can help with the loss of weight and support certain causes contributing to obesity, such as persistent inflammation. Specialists often consider that certain chronic diseases of proper digestive hygiene are easy to prevent.

People also feel more active and have restored vigor following detox. Since stress and contaminants impair the regular operation of the body, you might start feeling like your old self and bouncing back into good health.

Some Other Advantages of Detoxing for Digestion

Detox can also help in cleaning the large intestine or liver, where the healthy bacteria break down the food. In addition, colon cleansing assists in other stomach disorders, such as constipation and abnormal bowel movements. Therefore, it can also reduce the chances of colon cancer. By eating foods such as leafy greens and broccoli may help detoxify the colon, of course.

Digestive Problems and Detox Strategies

Be aware of what's going through your body when it comes to seeking treatment for stomach disorders that are perfect for your needs. For your digestive well-being, your dietary patterns, food nutrients, and detox remedies all play a role. For you, the right approach will also rely on your living style.

Many people consume more vegetables or nuts than products that are refined. Some use other foods to cleanse their bodies as laxatives. Natural remedies such as ginger or apple cider vinegar can help, for example, with negative symptoms. In fact, people use detox foods to remove contaminants from the body, varying from juice fasts to supplements or diuretics. Even some ready-made herbal cleansing mixes, sold in herbal stores, can be effective for cleansing the entire body or a particular area, such as the colon.

FASTING

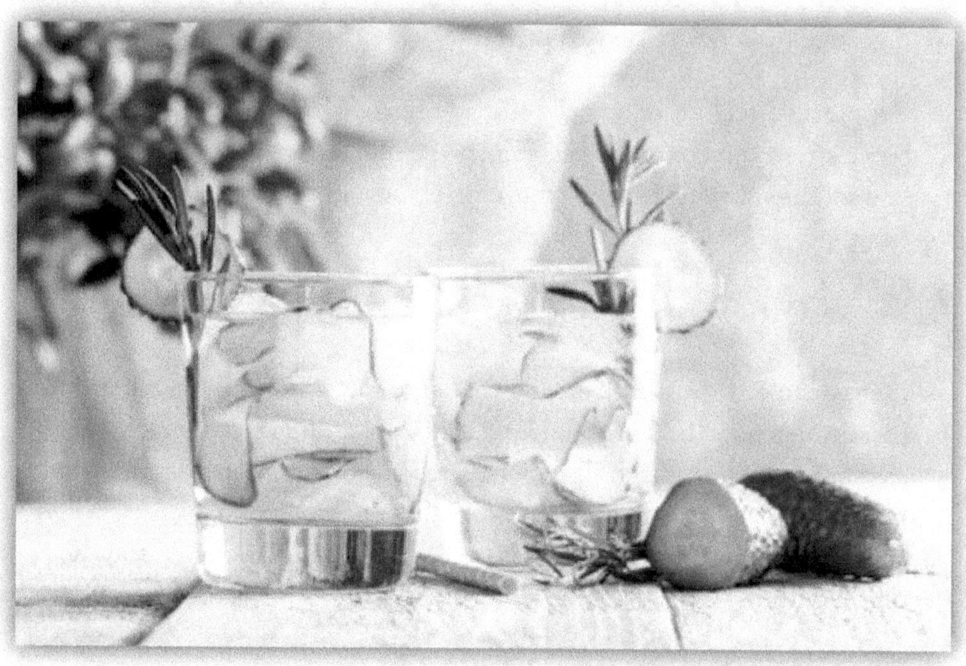

The best way to safely fast is the question on the lips of many. Before we delve into that, there is a need to paint a clearer picture of what fasting is. Self-restraint from food completely or partly for some motive is what is look upon as fasting. It can be dry or liquid. Surely, fasting maded with the use of vegetable juices and centrifuges, is the healthiest, most effective and easy way to follow a fast on an alkalizing basis. According to Dr. Alvenia Fulton, "The best juices are fresh juices made from your blender out of fresh fruits and vegetables, not from canned or frozen foods."

Before You Fast

Start fasting only when you are truly ready. You should never fast when your body is not ready; and if you feel hungry during a fast, you should eat. Take your time to get organized, and keep in mind that fasting is done in two stages to effectively cleanse your body. Firstly, you have to cleanse your body with natural herbs for at least five days before embarking on the actual fasting. In the meantime, you'll start lightening up your meals by increasing your vegetable consumption, eliminating harmful foods and drinking plenty of water.

Your body will give an indication to know when you are ready for the fast, and the indication you will have is during the cleansing phase with the herbs that, by detoxifying your body, will prepare it for the actual fast.

Why Should You Fast

If you want to know how to correct your body's discomforts, fasting will fix your body and keep you younger. The best method of fasting is to clean the body until there is no more hunger. When there is no hunger, you can fast as long as you like. You will become strong, addictions will be a distant memory, physical and mental abilities will improve. In fasting your tongue will become white and pasty (this is normal, it's the toxins leaking out); fast until your tongue turns red again, and fast until your breath and the smell of your body become "sweet" again. The body will also change its smell due to the removal of all the toxic waste in the body.

How to Prepare for Fasting

As stated above, your fasting should start with cleansing. Use different natural herbs for 3 to 5 days before starting your fast, be it a juice, a vegetable, or water fast. Take herbs first to remove some of the toxins and body waste. Most people have toxins that have been in their bodies since they were babies, so herbs are very important before any type of fasting. For example, the first time I tried fasting, the first days I could not stop go to the bathroom because I had many toxins coming out of me. And me, I really wasn't expecting that! But I was very glad to be rid of it, even though the feeling was provoking me discomfort at the time. On the other hand, I had never experienced anything like it before. And I wasn't even prepared for all that was waiting for me. I can tell you now, that these kinds of things don't happen anymore, and even when I get ready to do a new fast, it all happens smoothly, because my body has freed itself from the chronic toxic load.

How Long Should You Fast

Fasting is something very personal, and I recommend having a physical checkup and measurement of all values, to ensure that you are ready to do the fast. After that, starting a fast is a "journey", and the length and quality of the journey depends on our approach. Indicatively, I recommend that after cleansing your body with herbs, you continue your fast until your tongue is no longer "slick" (a sign that the toxins have left your body), you no longer feel tired, weak or nervous, and you feel rejuvenated. People around you will ask what you are doing; you will look younger. At that point, break the fast and gradually start eating again; A clean body maintains high performance even after fasting, both energetically and hormonally.

Fasting as the elixir of life

Experiencing the fast, you will conclude that what keeps us alive as beings is not food. What keeps us alive is the achievement of eliminating waste and toxins from our bodies. When we eat what nature has provided us, and in addition, we fast cleanse our body, our body and our mind will change and "reciprocate".

Our ancestors do not have prostate gland problems like the young men of nowadays. Our grandmothers as well did not lose their youthful factor as it is in today's world. In fact, my great-grandmother had twin babies at the age of 49, but this is unheard of in the 21st century despite all the medical discoveries. When we eat according to what nature has in store for us, we will stay healthy, live longer, and every pain in the body will vanish. Good health will ultimately triumph when we cleanse our bodies and stick to the right diet. On the other hand, "we are what we eat", but I would say... also what we don't eat.

Important factors related to fasting

The main contributors to self-sustainability, disease recovery, and quality of life are nutritional status. Obesity can result from overeating, dietary errors, or other various metabolic, genetic, and behavioral defects, causing both resistance of insulin and dysfunction of pancreatic beta cells and is, therefore, considered the foundation of diabetes type 2.

To promote weight loss, intermittent fasting, wherein people fast on sequential or alternating days, was being reported to prevent the development of diabetes type 2 and consequently boosted cardiovascular risk. Substantial evidence indicates that the imposition of fasting periods on laboratory animals enhances survival, promotes health, and decreases illness, including multiple morbidities with neurological cancer disorders and circadian rhythm disorders. Fasting is being used in religion from millennia. In those disciplines is usually carried out for three weeks. All Muslims worldwide fast during the daytime all over the Ramadan month, which is the 9th month of the Muslim calendar; this is considered one of the five critical pillars of Islam.

These fasting periods can reduce inflammation, amplify pro-inflammatory immune cells and cytokines, boost the levels of circulating lipids and glucose, and decrease blood pressure. Besides, experiments on humans and animals have indicated that the selection of fuel is changed, and metabolism efficiency is increased, whereas oxidative stress is decreased.

Some cardiac benefits are caused by random fasting, as indicated by animal models, such as raising heart rate and blood pressure, circulating triglycerides and cholesterol, and reducing intima-media carotid thickness. Besides, it enhances myocardial ischemia survival by anti-apoptotic, pro-angiogenic, and anti-remodeling impact.

Intermittent fasting also tends to be cardio protective, giving resistance to ischemic injury, to laboratory animals, in a way likely associated with a rise in adipokine adiponectin levels. Adiponectin is a distinctive adipokine that tends to have positive effects but also has circulation levels that are associated negatively with the composition of the body. Intermittent fasting, however, attenuates visceral fat levels and multiple specific adipokines, like IL-6, IGF-1, TNF-alpha, and leptin.

Although Ramadan fasting is compulsory for all the Muslims that value the religious atmosphere throughout the month of Ramadan, the Qur'an disallows from fasting those who are sick, traveling, expectant mothers, mothers during feeding, or females during their menstrual phase. In particular, fasting can be dangerous with diabetes as it could raise the incidence of postprandial hyperglycemia, dehydration, hypoglycemia, and thrombosis, both with and without diabetic ketoacidosis. Evaluating one's condition before embarking on a fasting journey is, therefore, highly recommended.

Benefits of Fasting

Fasting Promotes Blood Sugar Control

Intermittent fasting is believed to enhance blood sugar-lowering insulin hormone sensitivity and defend against fatty liver disease. Researchers have now revealed that mice often display lower fat cells in the pancreas on a fasting schedule. The researchers demonstrated, in their recent study, printed in a journal, the pathway through which fat cells in the pancreas would lead to the occurrence of diabetes type 2.

As a recognized and commonly occurring condition, the fatty liver was being extensively studied. Little is understood about the accumulation of fats in the pancreas caused by the extra weight and its impact on diabetes type 2. Work has now shown a high concentration of pancreatic fat cells in obese mice vulnerable to diabetes. Despite the extra weight, mice are immune to diabetes because of their genetic sequence with barely any pancreatic fats but instead had excess fat in the liver. The accumulation of fats external to the fat tissue, such as in the liver, bones, or even muscles, has a detrimental impact on these structures and the body.

Pancreatic Fat is Decreased by Intermittent Fasting

The team of experts split the diabetes-prone overweight animals into two categories: the first group was permitted to consume ad libitum — as much as they wished. The second group endured a random fasting routine: one day, the animals received an unlimited meal, and they were not fed at all the next day. The researchers noticed differences in the later five weeks. They concluded that the fat cells are accumulated in group 1 animals. Meanwhile, there are rarely any fat deposits in group 2 animals.

Fasting Enhances Heart Health

Heart health can be enhanced by fasting as it refines blood pressure, levels of cholesterol, and triglycerides.

Heart disease is recognized internationally as the leading cause of death, responsible for approximated 31.5% of deaths internationally. Among the most important ways to reduce, the risk of heart disease is to mix up the diet and lifestyle. Some studies have found that it can be incredibly helpful for heart health to integrate fasting into your routine.

Research showed that intermittent fasting for eight weeks decreases levels of "poor" LDL cholesterol by 25% and reduces blood triglycerides by 32%.

Another analysis of 110 overweight individuals demonstrated that, under medical supervision, fasting for three weeks substantially lowers blood pressure and blood triglyceride levels, total "bad" LDL cholesterol, and total cholesterol.

Furthermore, in one study of 4,629 individuals, fasting was associated with a reduced risk of coronary artery disorder and a slightly reduced risk of diabetes, a risk factor for heart disease.

Fasting Boosts Brain Function

New research shows that fasting can improve brain function by raising protein levels that encourage neuron growth.

The results suggest the treatment and prevention of age-related neurodegenerative diseases such as Alzheimer's disease are correlated with diabetes type. Researchers examined brain neurochemistry and brain activity of mice placed on intermittent fasting and normal eating. Many studies are conducted on neurodegenerative diseases underlying molecular and cellular processes. They have also thoroughly studied how fasting can increase the amount of energy in neurons and enable the brain to resist disease.

Earlier work indicates that fasting is a brain challenge that activates chemicals that encourage greater neuron efficiency and development. It can also have this effect by performing rigorous exercise.

One unique chemical shift potentially gives more energy to neurons and improves links to other neurons. Researchers noticed that fasting mice displayed a 50% rise in a chemical in the brain called BDNF (brain-derived neurotrophic factor), triggered by a surge in beta-hydroxybutyrate in the ketone body as fasting burns fat.

It is known that BDNF facilitates the development of new stem cell neurons, greater neuronal connections, and strengthens the synapses.

The fasted mice and the rise in BDNF showed increased alertness and activation in brain regions involved in learning and memory.

The cognitive advantages of fasting may originate from a rise in the number of nerve cell mitochondria due to increased levels of BDNF. Neurodegeneration has historically been associated with a deficiency or dysfunction of brain mitochondria.

Increasing the number of mitochondria in neurons will improve their ability to shape and sustain synapses and, therefore, likely increase the capacity for learning and memory.

Fasting Can Delay Aging and Increase Longevity

A molecule produced during fasting or calorie restriction has anti-aging effects on the vascular system, which could reduce the occurrence and severity of blood vessel-related diseases, such as cardiovascular disease, according to a study conducted by Georgia State University: The molecule, β-hydroxybutyrate.

The anti-aging molecule caused by fasting preserves young blood vessels. The results might help to avoid chronic age-related diseases like heart disease, cancer, and Alzheimer's.

Researchers have discovered that the molecule created during fasting can sustain our vascular system young and flexible.

In this study, researchers have practically nullified the symptoms of aging symptoms such as wrinkles and loss of hair in mice in a new analysis, and, in a brilliant new analysis, another group of scientists has succeeded in rejuvenating aging human cells. Fasting or reducing the intake of calories may generate then, this molecule that slows down vascular aging. Senescent cells can no longer multiply and divide.

Because this molecule is produced during caloric restriction or fasting, when people overeat or become obese, this molecule is probably suppressed, which would accelerate aging.

YOUR FOOD PANTRY

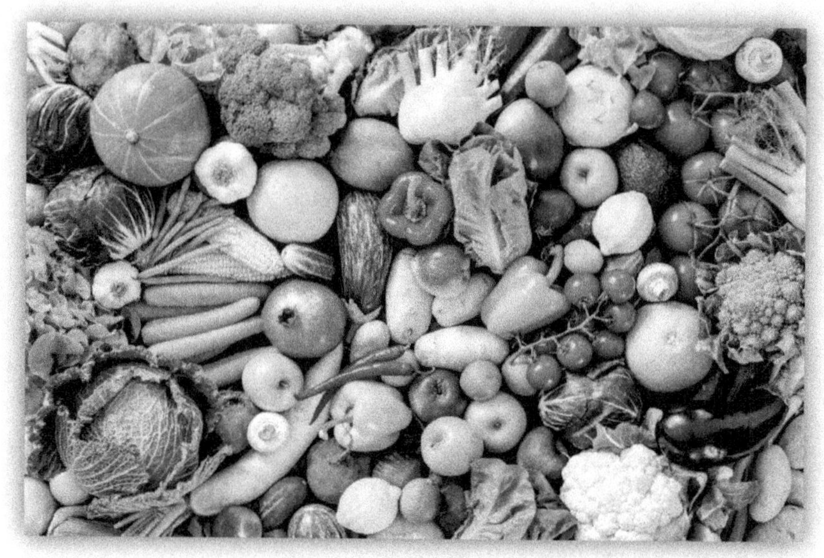

Approved Lists

Dr. Sebi created his diets from just live and raw food groups, virtually shutting out the rest of the food groups. He encouraged patients to consume more foods that are close to a raw vegan diet, such as, vegetables and fruits that are naturally grown, and whole grains. His line of thought was that the live and raw foods were electric, and they combat the acidic food waste produced in the body. Dr. Sebi compiled his food list he called "Electric Food List," he considered this best of his diets. This list continues to evolve and grow even after his demise.

For most people who eat out regularly, it can be challenging to abide by Dr. Sebi's food diets. It will be great for you to start approaching yourself for vegan diet meals by learning how to prepare such meals, using olive oil, wild rice, agave syrup, etc.

Dr. Sebi did not believe in calories or any kind of calculation on food. This is why his recipes do not include any calorie information. Just be sure to eat a varied diet, following the rules related to the stage you're in (if you're in detox, avoid grains, oils, nuts and seeds; if you're in maintenance, refer to the approved lists). By following the rules, you'll give your body adequate nutrition, including all the nutrients it needs for health, and it won't exceed its needs by putting on weight.

Vegetables

Dr. Sebi strongly advocates that people should consume non-genetically modified organism foods, which include seedless vegetables and fruits, or those modified to contain more nutrients than the natural state. He has a long, diverse list of vegetables, providing more options to make different unique meals. These are:

- Amaranth
- Avocado
- Arame
- Bell Pepper
- Cherry and Plum Tomato
- Mushroom apart from Shitake
- Chayote
- Cucumber
- Turnip Greens

- Dulse

- Dandelion Greens

- Hijiki

- Izote Flower and Leaf

- Kale

- Lettuce apart from Iceberg

- Wakame

- Nori

- Nopales

- Garbanzo Beans

- Onions

- Wild Arugula

- Olives

- Okra

- Zucchini

- Purslane Verdolaga

- Sea Vegetables

- Squash

- Tomatillo

- Watercress

Natural remedies and herbs

- Bilberry — Berry, and leaf (helps microcirculation)

- Bitter Melon — Fruit and seeds

- Bladderwrack — Whole herb (vitamin and mineral supplement)

- Blueberry— Fruit and leaf (eyes, bladder, microcirculation)

- Burdock — Root (blood and liver purifying, diuretic)

- Dandelion — Root and leaf (purifies blood and liver)

- Oregano - oil - (antiviral)

- Eucalyptus — Leaf

- Fenugreek — Seeds

- Fig — Fruit and leaf

- Guacos — Root

- Guinea Hen Weed {Anamu}— Whole plant

- Ginger — Root (fortifying, depurative)

- Huereque {Wereke} — Root

- Holy Basil — Leaf

- Irish Sea Moss — Whole Herb (vitamin and mineral supplement)

- Linden {Tila} — Flower and Leaf

- Mango — Fruit and Leaf

- Milk Thistle — Seeds

- Mulberry — Leaf

- Nettle — Leaf

- Nopal Cactus — Flat Stems

- Okra — Whole and Seeds

- Cactus {Prickly Pear} — Whole Fruit — Juice and Seeds

- Prodijiosa — Leaf

- Raspberry — Berry, and Leaf

- Black Walnut - (kills pests)

- Absinthe (kills pests)

- Sage - Leaf

- Elderberry (strengthens the body against infections)

- Mullein - (removes mucus in the small intestine)

- Sage — Leaf

- Seville {Sour Orange} — Fruit

- Sour Soup — Fruit and Juice

Natural Herbal Teas

- Chamomile
- Red Raspberry

- Elderberry
- Tila
- Fennel
- Burdock
- Ginger

Grain

- Wild Rice
- Fonio
- Quinoa
- Rye
- Amaranth
- Spelt
- Tef
- Kamut

Nut and Seeds

- Raw Sesame Seeds
- Walnuts
- Brazil Nuts
- Hemp Seeds
- Raw Tahini

Oils

- Avocado Oil

- Coconut Oil
- Grape seed Oil
- Hempseed Oil
- Olive Oil
- Sesame Oil

Flavors and Seasoning

- Achiote
- Bay Leaf
- Basil
- Cloves
- Cayenne
- Dill
- Habanero
- Oregano
- Onion Powder
- Pure Sea Salt
- Savory
- Sweet Basil
- Sage
- Thyme
- Tarragon

Fruit List

While Dr. Sebi proposes a wide range of vegetables, he places many restrictions on fruits. Despite this restriction, fruits have a diverse range of lists to choose from including all varieties of berries apart from cranberries that are human-made. These are:

- Apples
- Berries
- Bananas
- Cherries
- Currants
- Elderberry
- Cantaloupe
- Dates
- Figs
- Grapes
- Limes
- Melons
- Mango
- Orange
- Plums
- Papayas
- Prunes
- Peaches
- Pears
- Prickly Pear
- Raisins
- Sour soups
- Soft Jelly Coconut
- Tamarind

Sweeteners and Sugars

- 100% Pure Agave Syrup From Cactus

- Date Sugar From Dried Dates

Guidelines for Dr. Sebi's Approved Foods and Herbs

- You should drink two liters of water daily, preferably natural spring water.

- Plastic and rubber are toxic materials. Do not take water (or food) from a disposable container where you find remnants or traces of toxic toxins, but prefer glass containers.

- If you are taking pharmaceutical drugs, take Dr. Sebi's product an hour prior.

- Strict adherence to Dr. Sebi's nutritional guidelines guarantees the best result in disease reversal.

- No fish, no alcohol, no animal products, no hybrid foods, and no dairy.

- Consume only the above-approved grains.

- Many of the approved grains are sold in health food stores as bread, pasta, cereal, or flour.

- Dr. Sebi's products work for 14 days within the body, as it still releases therapeutic properties.

- Do not make use of the microwave, and it kills the food.

- No consumption of seedless or canned fruits.

Prohibited Foods

Foods that are not written below approved Dr. Sebi diet list is prohibited from being consumed, some of such foods are:

- Seedless Fruits

- Canned Fruits or Vegetables

- Fish

- Dairy

- Poultry

- Red Meat

- Fortified Foods

- Soy Products

- Wheat

- Alcohol

- Processed foods, including restaurant foods and take-outs

- Yeast enhanced food

- Food made with baking powder

- Sugar apart from agave syrup and date sugar

- Eggs

Dr. Sebi's Method of Classifying Foods

He classified the foods list into six classes. These classes are:

1. Living foods

2. Raw foods

3. Hybrid foods

4. Dead foods

5. Genetically modified foods

6. Drugs

Living Foods

These foods are not dead without consuming them, which means that only inside the body they undergo a transformation, but before that they are alive and full of energy. These live foods don't produce toxic components even when left to ferment.

More so, living foods do not undergo destruction when they are not in their environment. The materials required for digestion are embedded in living food, which contains almost the same PH as water (PH 7). Examples are green vegetables, fruits that ripen from the tree, grain, and many others.

Raw Foods

These are living foods with undergone processing and they are undercooked. They are foods that are dried with the use of direct sunlight.

These foods also contain many components needed for the digestion process and are spoiled within a short time if not adequately dried. Examples are dried fruits and vegetables, vegetables that roasted, fermented fruit juice, and many others.

Dead Foods

These are foods that, when fermented, become toxic, and have a prolonged life span. They are overdone and over-processed foods. Examples are deep-fried foods, synthetic foods, alcohols, sugars. Foods that have no energy intake, only a toxic load.

Hybrid Foods

They are foods that are not naturally grown but are cross-pollinated. The vitamins and mineral levels cannot be quantified, and they cannot be produced in the wild. Hybrid foods are mostly sugars that are not recognized by the digestive system.

Genetically Modified Foods (Gmo)

These are food improved by the man with the use of genetics. They mostly damage immunity in humans. These foods form an abnormal attitude in humans and cause genetic consequences in the body. Examples are grown hastily, weather-resistant foods such as corn, yeast, brown rice, and many others.

Drugs

Under the definition of drugs fall also things you don't expect, and that is all those foods that not only create damage but also addiction. Many drugs are dangerous and harmful to the body. They are incredibly toxic and acidic. Most of them are extracted and are synthetic. Most of them are chemically extracted and synthetic. They alter the brain structure, are addictive, and destroy the immune system, in addition to damaging numerous organs. Examples are cocaine, sugar (well yes, it is a drug), all prescription drugs, heroin, and many others. Vibrationally they are the deadliest elements we introduce into the body and act as true "energy vampires".

DR. SEBI APPROVED HERBS: THEIR BENEFITS, DOSAGE, HOW TO PREPARE AND USE THEM

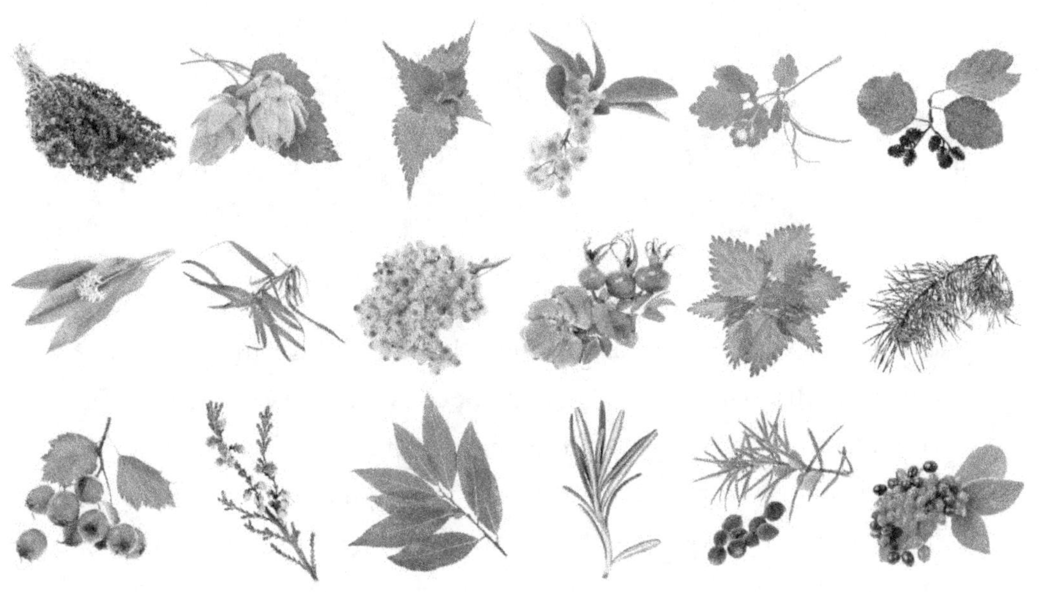

Irish Sea Moss

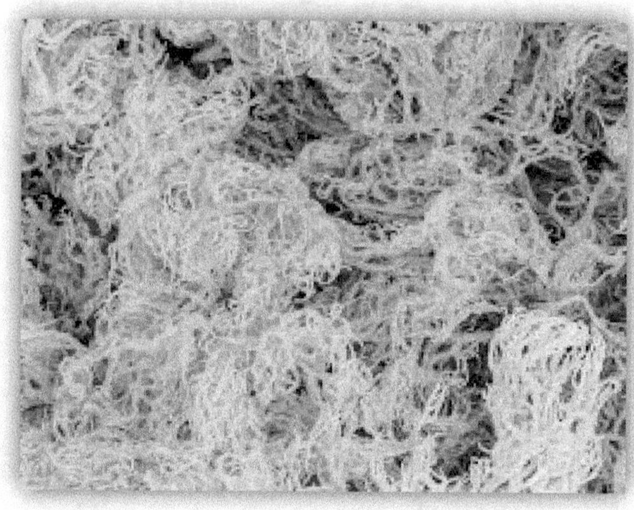

Irish Sea Moss is red algae that belong to the family of Florideophytes that grows on the rocky parts of the Atlantic coast of various countries like the British Isles, Ireland, Jamaica, Scotland, etc. One amazing fact about this herb that makes Dr. Sebi recommends it for cleansing and revitalizing the body system is that it contains about 92 out of the 102 minerals that the body needs to be healthy. Some of the minerals that it contains are iodine, selenium, calcium, bromine, zinc, iron, phosphorus, potassium, etc.

Benefits of Consuming Irish Sea Moss

- It helps to heal and boost the immune defense system

- It helps to treat and prevent hyperthyroidism and boosts the functionalities and health of the thyroid gland

- It helps to soothe joint pain and swelling of the joint and treat arthritis

- It helps to enrich the overall mood and reduce fussiness

- It helps to combat infections caused by viruses and bacteria

- It helps to treat and prevent digestive and respiratory tract disorders

- It helps to treat and prevent various skin disorders like acne, skin wrinkling and alleviates inflammation

Side Effects of Consuming Irish Sea Moss Are

- Spewing

- Burning sensation or itching (mouth and throat)

- Fever

- Stomach irritation

- Nausea

Bladderwrack

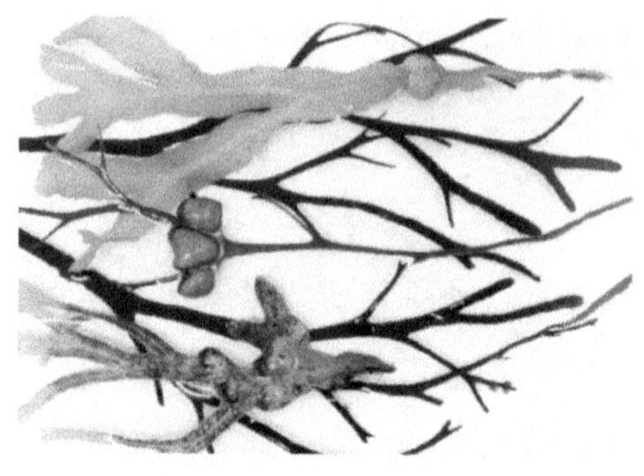

Bladderwrack (Fresh)

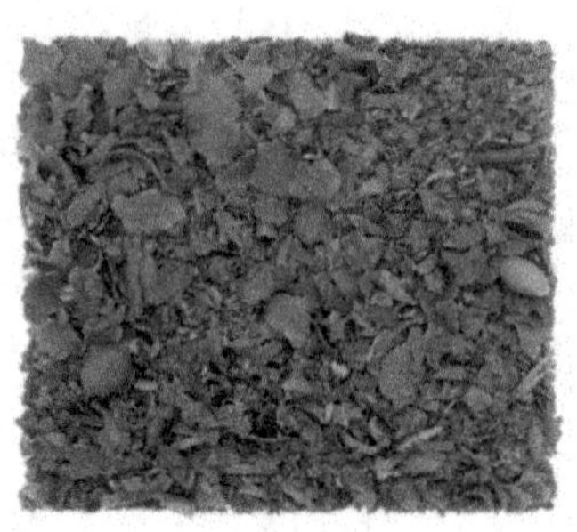

Bladderwrack (Dried)

Bladderwrack is found on the coasts of the western Baltic Sea, the North Sea, and the Pacific and Atlantic Oceans. It is high in iodine — a key substance for thyroid health.

Uses: Used to take care of many thyroid ailments, e.g. underactive thyroid, outsized thyroid Gland, and potassium deficiency. It's also utilized for heartburn, arthritis, bronchitis, obesity, arteriosclerosis, digestive disorders, blood cleansing, emphysema, urinary tract disorders, constipation as well as nervousness. Other uses include boosting the immune system and increasing energy.

How to Use: Bladderwrack might be consumed completely, taken as a tea, or even blended with sea turtles from beverages and smoothies. To make tea, then combine 1 teaspoon per cup of warm spring water, and then allow to sit for 15 minutes prior to drinking. This may be taken one or two times every day.

Caution: Bladderwrack may potentially contain high levels of potassium, which might worsen some thyroid issues, so avoid protracted high or used doses.

Cascara Sagrada

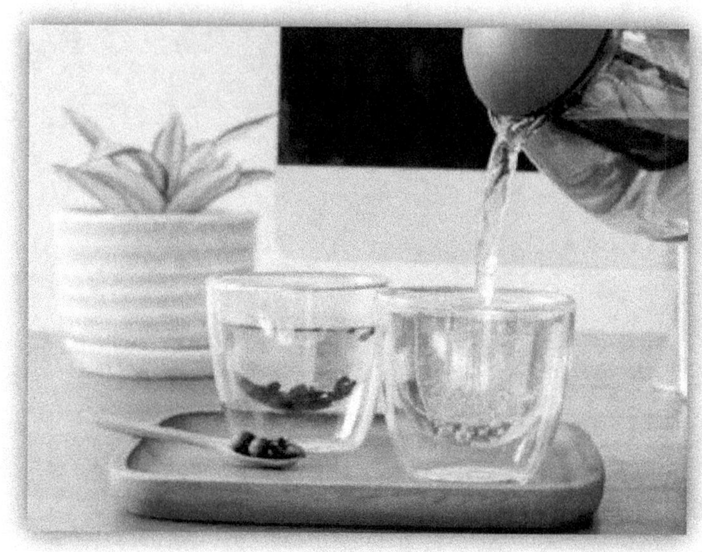

Considered a high All-natural laxative by herbalists. It's supposed to be the best herb for colon cleansing accessible. Cascara Sagrada is proven to serve as a natural antibiotic in the intestines when taken internally. It's been used to eliminate gastrointestinal ailments such as worms.

How it Functions: Cascara Sagrada will cause a bowel movement over eight to 12 hours taking a dose. It induces muscular contraction in the gut, which helps move stool throughout the gut. Additionally stimulates the liver/pancreas secretion.

Cascara Sagrada increases the secretion of bile in the gallbladder. Because of this property, it's been used to divide and prevent gallstones.

Key benefits: Laxative for constipation, therapy for hepatitis, liver disorders, and cancer. A colon cleaner thought to enhance the muscular tone of the colon walls.

Other Applications: It is believed to ease the strain and pain associated with hemorrhoids and anal fissures too (however this claim is just supported by traditional use).

Taste: It does not taste great.

How to Utilize: Cascara Sagrada will generally cause a bowel movement within 12 hours, so it is Ideal to take it at night in order that in the morning it is simpler to use the bathroom.

Caution/Side Outcomes: This can cause laxative dependence since the intestines start to adapt to these anthraquinones and be able to operate by themselves. Please refrain from accepting it for more than two weeks without needing a rest (at least two days). Don't advise.

Drinking this and then heading out for a very long amount of time in which you must use a toilet in somebody else's home.

Lilly of the Valley

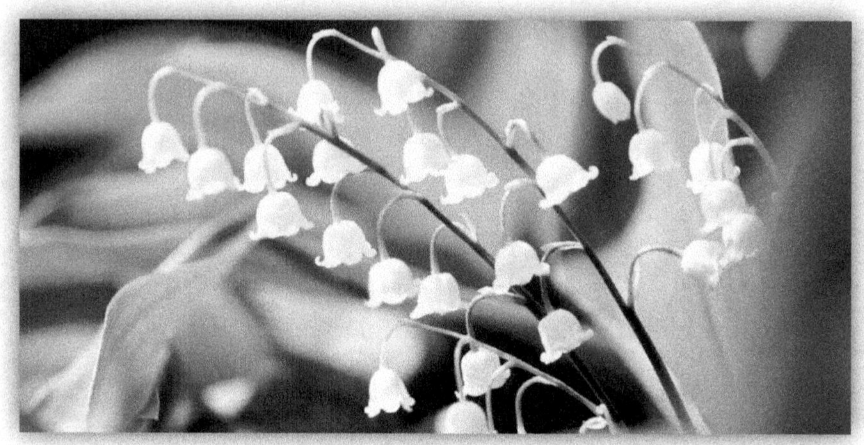

The Lilly-of-the-Valley plant is also known as the May Lily, and it can be found in forests, woods, valleys, and woodland edges. The flower is a pale pink color with four petals. Flowers bloom from April to June but they have a strong unpleasant odor. The leaves are heart-shaped and have a long stem above them.

It is rich in iron, fluorine, and potassium phosphate. It can be used as a diuretic, for kidney stones, as a cardiac tonic, and to address central nervous system disorders.

Santa Maria

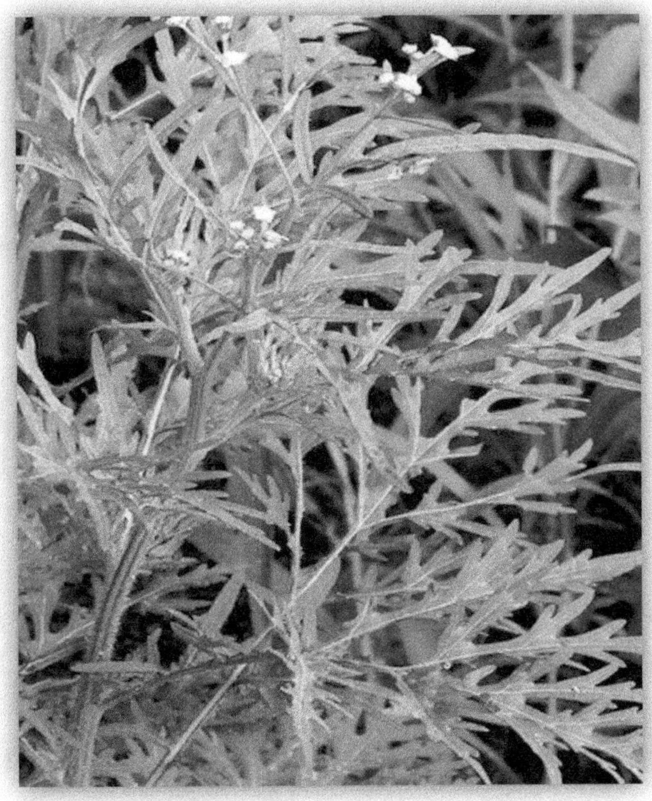

Recent studies show that this herb still holds many health benefits. Santa Maria is rich in minerals and vitamins and contains many other vital components, such as sesquiterpene lactones, sesquiterpenes (camphor), and volatile oil. These properties help this herb treat problems such as anxiety, arthritis, stress, migraines, inflammation, blood pressure, and blood clots.

If you have heart problems, Santa Maria will help you too. It reduces the risk of having atherosclerosis, stroke, and heart attack. In fact, it reduces the production of prostaglandins that cause serious cardiovascular problems.

Remember that this is not a perfect herb because some side effects can also cause respiratory and dermatitis problems in humans. However, its advantages always outweigh its disadvantages. They are beneficial for many uncontrollable illnesses.

Other benefits include:

- Santa Maria treats coughs
- Cures joint pain and migraine
- Lessens painful menstruation and arthritis pains
- Cures hair fall and respiratory problems
- Used in the treatment of fever and cancer
- Cures appetite issues and dermatitis
- Cures blood clots
- Used to lessen stress and anxiety
- Cures inflammation, bruises, and swelling
- Used the treatment of breathing difficulties, blood pressure, and headaches

Prodijiosa

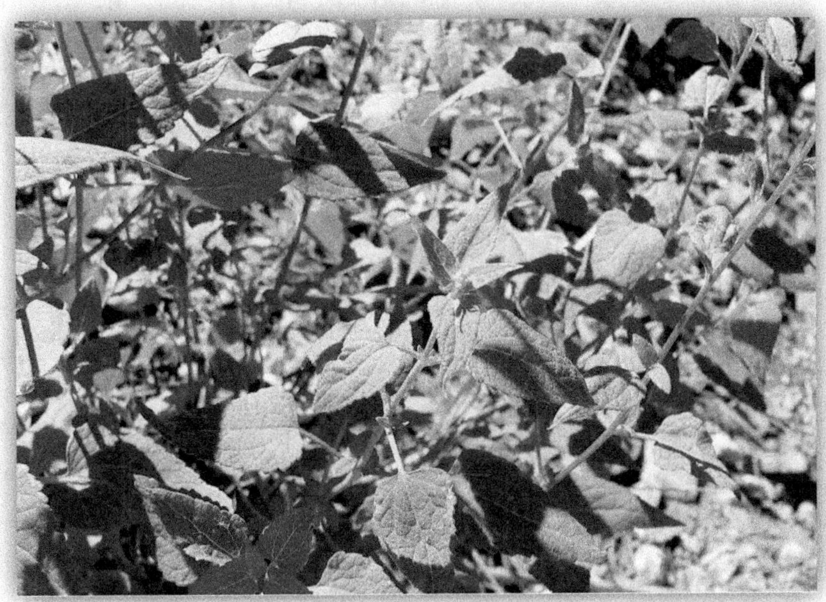

This really is a dark green bushy herb with leaves around the top side and a greyish purple color on the bottom. It develops as large as 5 feet. The flowers on this plant include a pure white color to a yellowish shade and may be seen growing in clusters. This perennial plant could be found flowering almost throughout the year.

Prodigiosa is frequently talked about as being correlated with all the dark arts because it had been used in voodoo for part of their rituals. However, this herb is not difficult to cultivate and develops just too in a plant pot. Its medicinal advantages shouldn't be overlooked and by developing this herb into your garden, you're never too much from a new cup of herbal tea.

Key Benefits: Prodigiosa arouses pancreas secretion, reduces blood glucose, and enhances fat digestion in the gall bladder. Helps with gut digestion, supports healthy kidney function, helps maintain Wholesome Glucose Levels, and supports a healthy immune system

Uses: Immune system, Gallbladder, and Pancreas, immune system health, reduces blood glucose, and is valuable for individuals with diabetes.

Taste: it's quite bitter in flavor.

You may think of this as a bad thing but when it comes to digestion, bitter is better.

How to Utilize: Take as a tea or in capsule form. Once consumed as a tea, then the herb produces lactic acid, which assists stomach digestion. Make a tea by brewing leaves (fresh or dried) in warm spring water. Since the sour flavor of these leaves, you may add date syrup into it. This tea may be taken twice each day.

Caution: Effects unwanted unknown.

Lavender

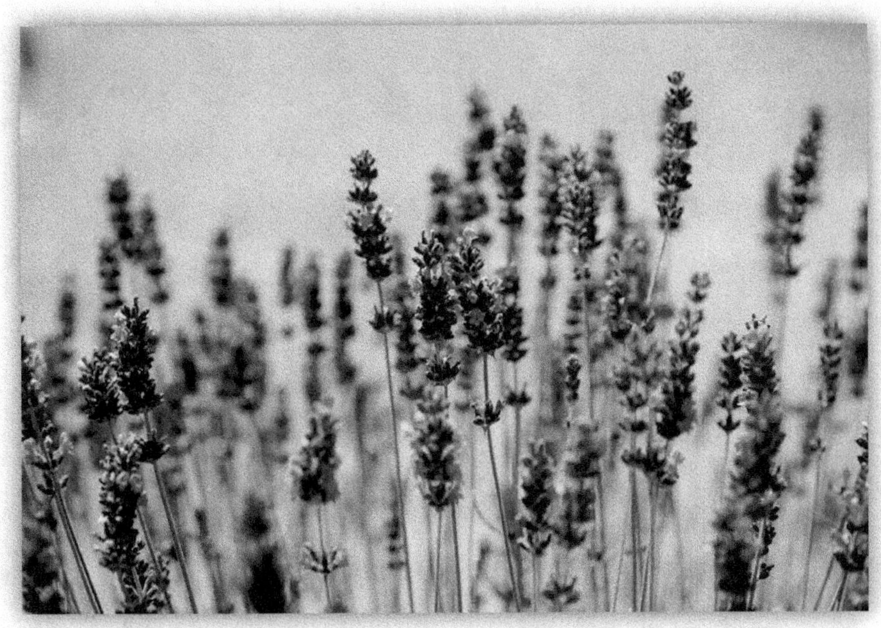

This herb has natural anti-seizure medicinal constituents that are capable of preventing convulsion. It also has a huge amount of analgesic property that provides instant relief of muscular pain, headache or one-sided headache (migraine), and joint pain.

It is a calming plant, now universally recognized. Its essential oils act directly on the nervous system, giving immediate relief.

Lavender oil contains antibacterial, antimicrobial, antiseptic, and anti-inflammatory components. It is essential in fighting baldness, increasing hair growth, and improves hair health. His oil helps in fighting hair and scalp problems such as head lice, dandruff, dry scalp, and many other scalp infections. The constant use of this oil assists in preventing hair from falling off and facilitates rapid hair growth. You can use this oil by applying it to your scalp and hair and massage it very well to ensure penetration of the oil on the hair.

Sarsaparilla

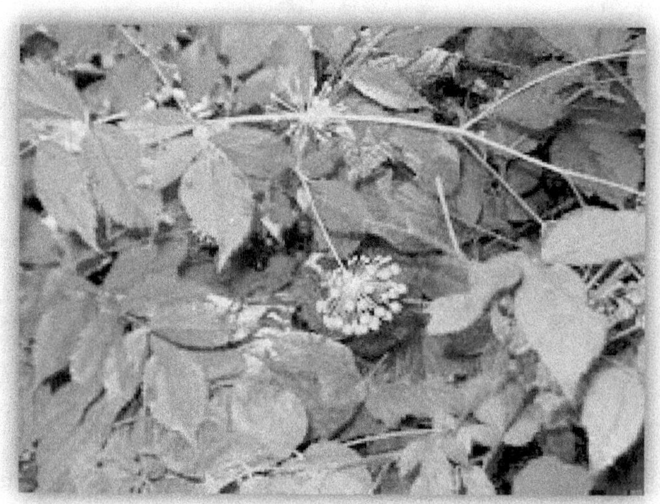

Sarsaparilla is a tropical wood climbing vine that belongs to the genus Smilax family. It is very rich in iron, calcium, phosphate, sarsaponin steroid, flavonoid, etc. body needs to speed up the healing and recovery process. Late Dr. Sebi recommended sarsaparilla as a revitalizing herb because of its potency to fast-track healing and recovery process.

Benefits of Consuming Sarsaparilla

- It binds the endotoxins responsible for the lesions in psoriasis patients and eliminates them from the body system

- It helps treat and prevent health issues caused by inflammation like joint pain, swelling of any parts of the body, arthritis, rheumatoid, etc.

- It helps to soothe and heals sexually transmitted diseases such as syphilis, herpes, gonorrhea, etc.

- It helps to treat and prevent leprosy

- It helps to destroy and prevent cancerous cells from mutating

- It helps to protect, and reverse damages done to the liver to function correctly

- It helps to make the body absorb nutrients and other herbs quickly etc.

How to Prepare Sarsaparilla Root Tea Kindly Take the Following Steps:

- Harvest some sarsaparilla plant roots and wash them under running water to remove all the dirt that accompanied them from the soil

- After washing it, pill off the outer skin, chop it into smaller pieces, and dry it in a well-ventilated place (indoors) for at least seven days (ensure you turn the drying root daily for the 7 days until it is completely dried)

- Once it is dried, store it in a paper bag or cardboard box. (Ensure you don't keep it in a plastic container, as it will get mold)

- Measure 1teaspoon of the dried chopped Sarsaparilla root, add it to your saucepan, and add 8 ounces of water. Boil it for 15-20 minutes

- Strain it using a strainer. You are done!

- For the dosage, consume 1cup (8ounce) 3 times daily

Contribo

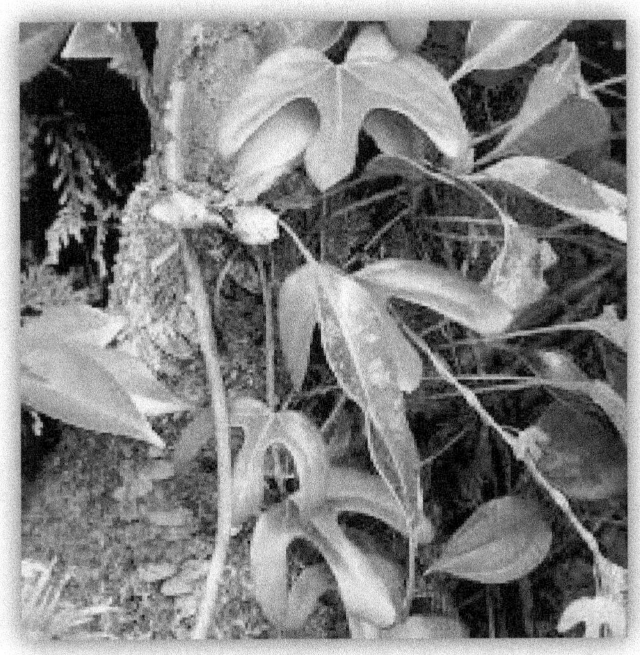

Contribo is a vine plant from the family of Aristolochiaceae. Dr. Sebi recommends it as a revitalizing herb because of its potency in rejuvenating the loss of energy that the body must have lost due to the disease, enrich mood, fight fatigue, boost appetite, etc.

Benefits of Consuming Contribo

- It helps to boost energy and stamina levels.

- It helps to enrich mood and relieve fatigue and depression.

- It helps to enhance and boost the circulatory system and increase appetite.

- It helps to combat delayed menstruation and fast track it.

- It helps enhance the health of the digestive system and gallbladder and relieves constipation.

- It helps to treat and prevent kidney disorders, dissolves kidney stones, and enhances kidney health.

- It helps to treat, dissolves bladder stones, and relieve uterine complaints.

- It helps to boost the immune defense system and also, calm and heal the immune system.

- It helps treat and prevent various diseases such as flu, stomach irritation, indigestion, colds, non-insulin-dependent diabetes, etc.

How to Prepare Contribo Tea or Infusion Kindly Take the Steps Below:

- Harvest some fresh vine of contribo, wash it, and dry it.

- Once it is dried, chop it into smaller pieces or order it online and it will come dried and chopped.

- Measure 1-2 teaspoons of contribo and add it to your saucepan.

- Pour 8-16 ounces of water and add it to the saucepan where the contribo vine is.

- Boil the mixture for 10-15 minutes.

- After boiling it, strain it.

-    For the dosage, take 1-2cups of contribo tea 2 times per day (preferably, morning and night).

-    Alternatively, if you have the fresh vine, wash it and soak it in boiling water for 24 hours.

-    For the dosage, ½ cups per week.

Hydrangea

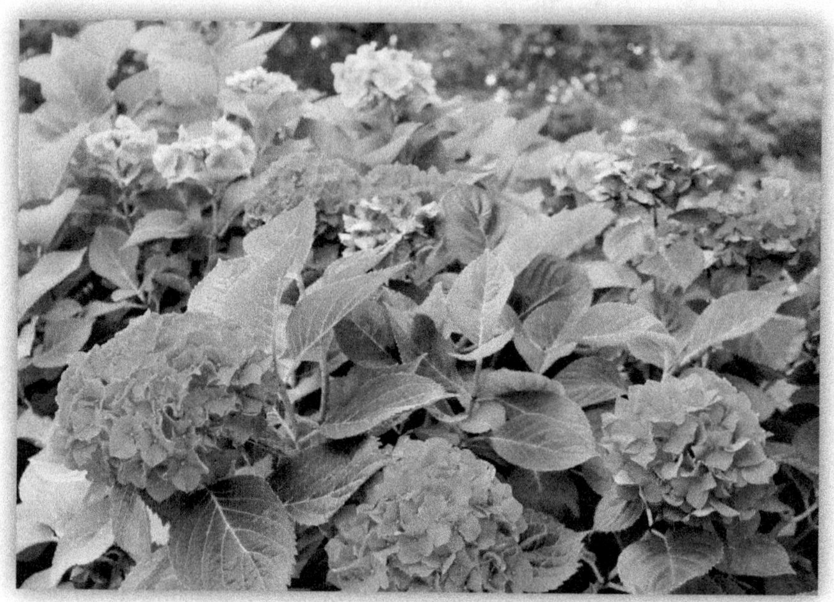

Hydrangea herb's roots contain many nutrients and phytochemicals such as zinc, selenium, and calcium. For this reason, Dr. Sebi used them to treat many health problems. Several people also try to use hydrangea leaves too, which is something that Dr. Sebi did not recommend because the leaves contain toxic substances. Hydrangea leaves should never be consumed either for medical or fun purposes.

Other benefits include:

- Treat wounds, sore muscles, burn, and sprain.
- It also helps in curing rheumatoid arthritis.
- Aids in treating inflammatory bowel disease.
- Treats multiple sclerosis.

- One can use this herb for treating chronic chest pains as well.

- Used to cure urinary tract problems and autoimmune disorders.

Purlsane

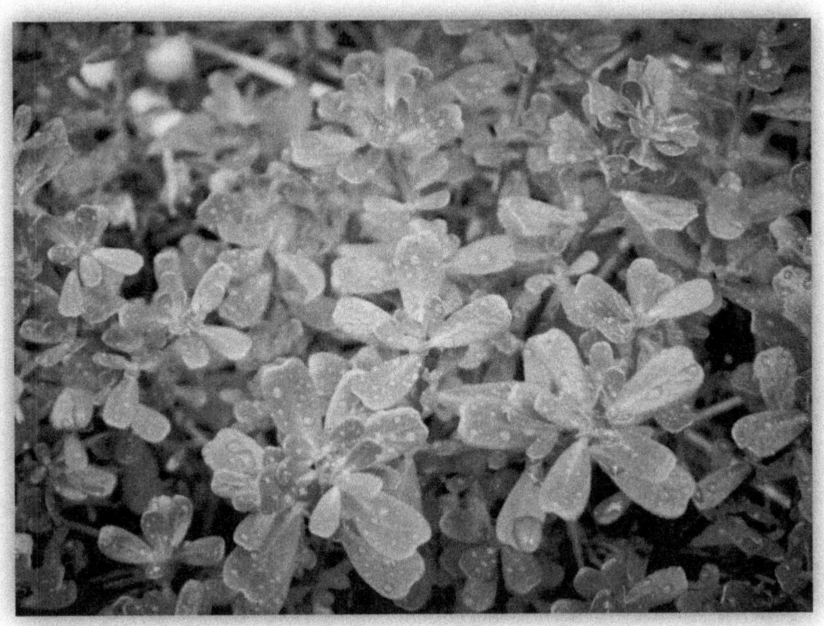

This plant is known in the UK as Marsh Lavender. The Purlsanes are named so because they grow in wet places or marshes. It is also called Sweet Lavender or Sea Lavender. The leaves have a very strong woody smell to them due to the oils contained within them, but the flowers have no odor at all.

Here are the key gains that you can benefit from taking this herb:

- Super rich in omega fatty acids
- Acts as an antioxidant

- Help with weight loss
- Improvement of gastrointestinal disorders
- Strengthening of the teeth and bones
- Improvement in blood circulation

Sage

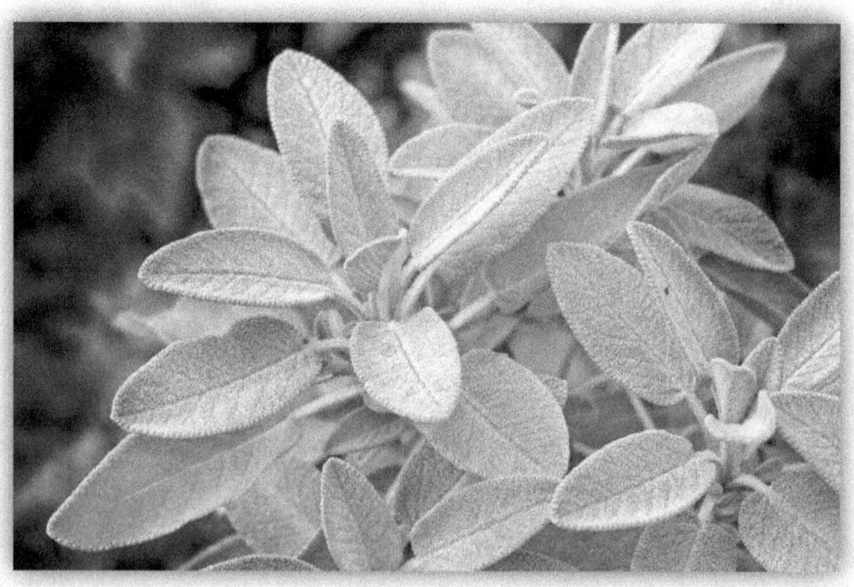

Dr. Sebi, plus several lab tests have confirmed the tremendous nutritional value of sage. One tablespoon of sage contains 43% vitamin K, and that is just the exact amount our body needs to function correctly. It is also an excellent source of vitamin E, vitamin C, vitamin

A, calcium, iron, magnesium, and fiber. It is also found that sage contains B-vitamins, such as riboflavin. Besides, they play an essential role in sustaining our body as a well-aligned machine.

When the right dosage is consumed, it can facilitate the treatment of inflammation, boosting female fertility, increasing memory retention, neutralizing free radicals, preventing gastric spasms, strengthening the immune system, preventing Alzheimer's disease, improving bone health, curing issues like arthritis and gout, managing diabetes and treatment of snake bites.

Other benefits include:

- Sage is antiseptic, antioxidant, and antibacterial.

- It is an excellent source of vitamin A, vitamin C, vitamin E, iron, calcium, magnesium, and fiber.

- It also treats conditions such as a weak immune system, arthritis, Alzheimer's, inflammation, and diabetes.

Red Clover

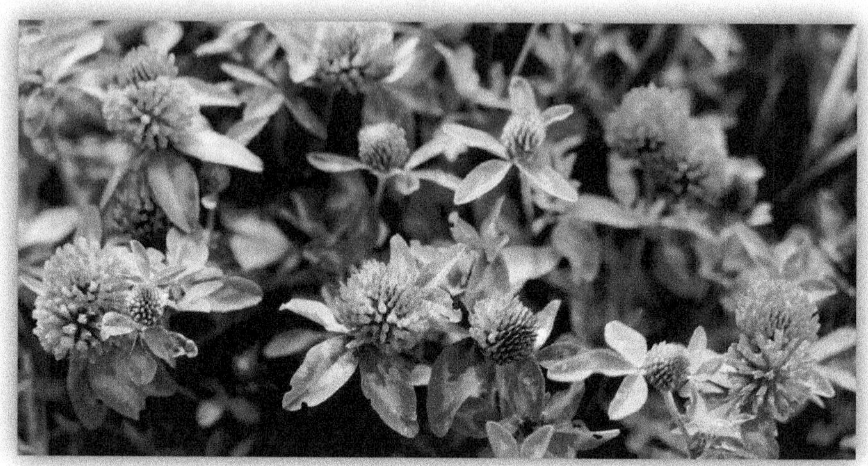

Red Clover is a low-growing annual plant that grows about 2-4 feet tall. It produces yellow flowers in March, April and May. These are followed by red-brown seed pods that reach around 1/2 inch in length. Red Clover is typically found in grasslands and open areas near forests or meadows.

Red clover active ingredients include:

- Phenolic glycosides
- Flavonoids
- Salicylates
- Coumarins
- Cyanogenic glycosides
- Mineral acids

Only the flowers have therapeutic properties and it's best to harvest them during flowering.

Effect it has on the body:

- Alterative
- Antispasmodic
- Diuretic
- Anti-inflammatory
- Oestrogenic properties

Traditionally, red clover was used for skin complaints; and to treat coughs and bronchitis but in the 1930s, it was recommended to treating certain types of cancer, e.g. breast, ovarian, and lymphatic. Unfortunately, after the boom of the pharmaceutical industry in the 1960s, red clover is no longer considered an effective cancer treatment. Still, many holistic doctors prescribe it as an anti-cancer therapy.

6 Ways to Use Red Clover Flowers.

1. **Fresh flowers**

   Crushed fresh flowers may be applied to insect bites and stings.

2. **Tincture**

   Take internally for skin problems like psoriasis and eczema.

3. **Compress**

   Use for arthritic pains and gout.

4. **Eyewash**

Use about 6-12 drops of tincture in about half an ounce (20 ml) spring water for a well-strained infusion for conjunctivitis or a full eyebath.

5. Douche

Use the infusion for vaginal itching.

6. Syrup

The syrup is an effective treatment for stubborn, dry coughs.

Blessed Thistle

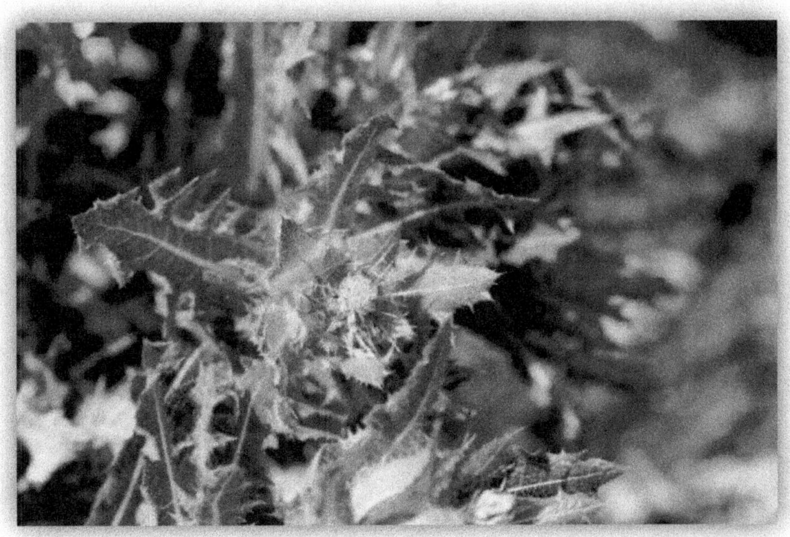

Blessed thistle is a medicinal plant that has been used since at least the Middle Ages. It is also known as "St. Benedict's thistle" or "holy thistle." It is brewed to make a medicinal tea and contains tannins. Traditionally it has been used to cure coughs and colds as well as digestive problems. A blessed thistle can also come in the form of a capsule.

The following are the benefits of using this medicinal herb:

- It promotes digestive health

- It is antimicrobial

- It is anti-inflammatory

- It protects the liver and kidney

- Stimulates appetite

- It is antibacterial

- It is helpful for stomach upset

- It stimulates milk supply

- It shrinks inflamed tissues

- It helps in treating arthritis, jaundice, and fevers

Valerian

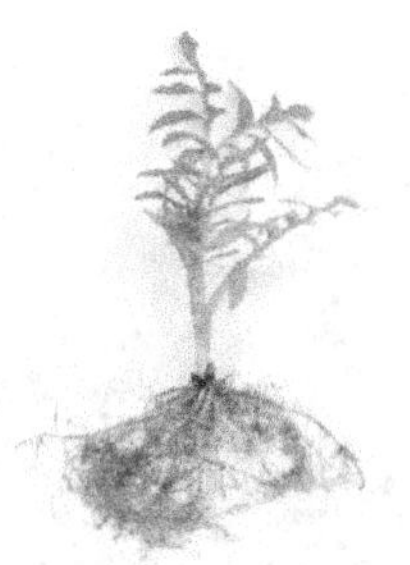

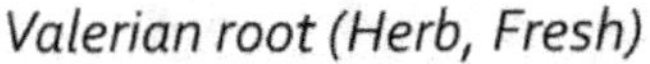

Valerian root (Herb, Fresh)

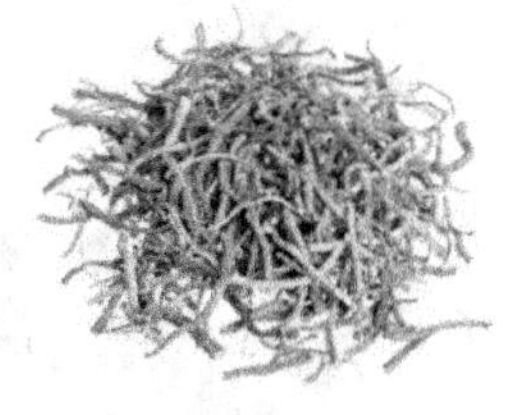

Valerian root (Herb, Dried)

An ancient remedy for anxiety, stress, nervous asthma, hysterical states, hypochondria, headaches, and stomach upsets. You can use it for hypertension caused by stress.

The properties of the officinal plant are due to the fact that the root is a real concentrate of chemical molecules, characterized by molecules having sedative, calming, antioxidant and antibacterial actions.

Valerian is used as a sedative and has also an important action as a calming agent.

Of the valerian plant is used the root, which can be used in infusion in order to obtain herbal teas with sedative action.

It is useful for:

- states of anxiety
- digestive difficulties
- inflammations of the mucosa of the stomach and of the first part of the intestine (duodenum) and of the last one (colon)
- topical inflammations such as erythema or acne.

Blue Vervain

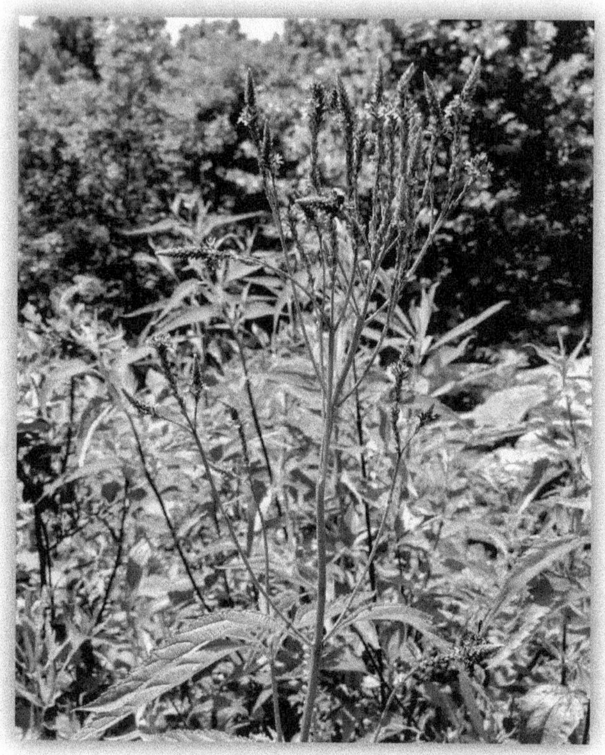

In pre-Christian England, vervain was considered a sacred herb. The ancient Romans also considered it sacred and used it to purify their homes and temples. It was regularly used in magic and ritual.

Blue vervain active ingredients include:

- Volatile oil
- Bitter glycosides
- Tannins

Dr. Sebi valued this herb very much and prescribed it for many conditions.

Medicinal properties of blue vervain:

- Relaxant tonic
- Promotes milk flow
- Stimulates labor
- Promotes sweating
- Nervine
- Sedative
- Antispasmodic
- Liver stimulant
- Laxative
- Uterine stimulant
- Urinary cleanser
- Fever remedy
- Bile stimulant.

Aerial parts should be gathered in summer while flowering. Vervain is usually taken internally but can be used topically as well.

Ways to use vervain:

- Infusion

Take for insomnia, nervous tension, or in case of fever to encourage sweating. Can also be used as a liver stimulant to improve appetite and digestion. If sipped during the labor, it will encourage contractions and if taken during lactation, will stimulate milk flow.

- Tincture

Use for depression, as a stimulant for liver, nervous exhaustion, or for poor digestion. It can be used in combination with other urinary herbs for stones and conditions related to excess uric acid.

* Poultice

Apply to muscle sprains, insect bites, and bruises.

* Ointment

Use on skin problems such as eczema or wounds. Can also be used for neuralgia.

* Mouthwash

You can use the infusion for spongy gums, or mouth ulcers.

Caution: Avoid the herb in pregnancy. This is because it stimulates the uterus. However, it may be taken during labor as it stimulates contractions.

Burdock Root

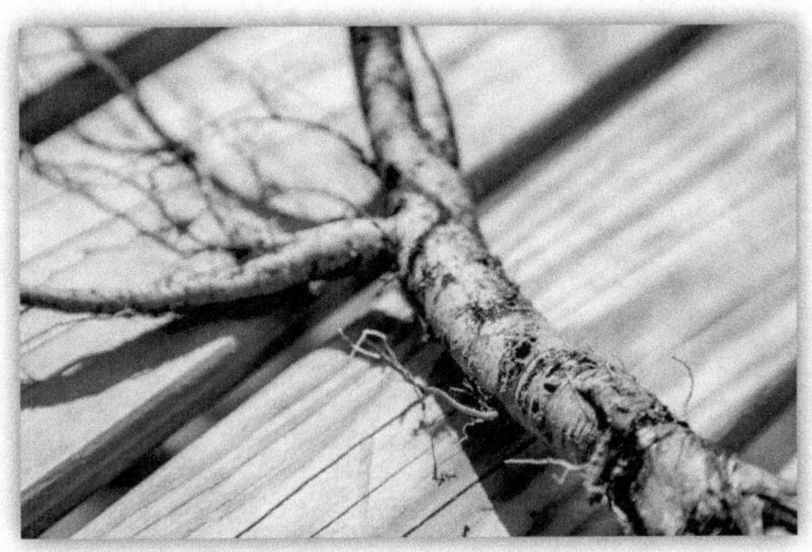

<u>Burdock Root comprises all 102 minerals, which form the human body in trace quantities.</u>

Key Benefits: Assists with indigestion, joint pain, detoxifying the liver, and balancing hormones. Helps improve skin quality, decrease inflammation, and reduce blood glucose levels. USES: Heal insomnia, cancer, gastrointestinal ailments, joint pain, arthritis, kidney infections, complications of syphilis, & skin ailments such as psoriasis. May assist with gout, thyroid health, bladder ailments + kidney & gallbladder stones.

Taste: Getting a nutty sweetness and taste

How to Use: Blend it with Dandelion Root to get a great "java" or into Perrier + Date Syrup to create a "beer." I love to blend it with other herbs to provide me a nutrient increase. Since Sarsaparilla is greatest in iron and behaves as a magnet for the rest of the minerals, I blend them frequently (typically, with a 3rd herb which rounds out the taste (such as Linden Flower).

Caution: If you've got a Bleeding disease, burdock may increase bleeding.

Eyebright

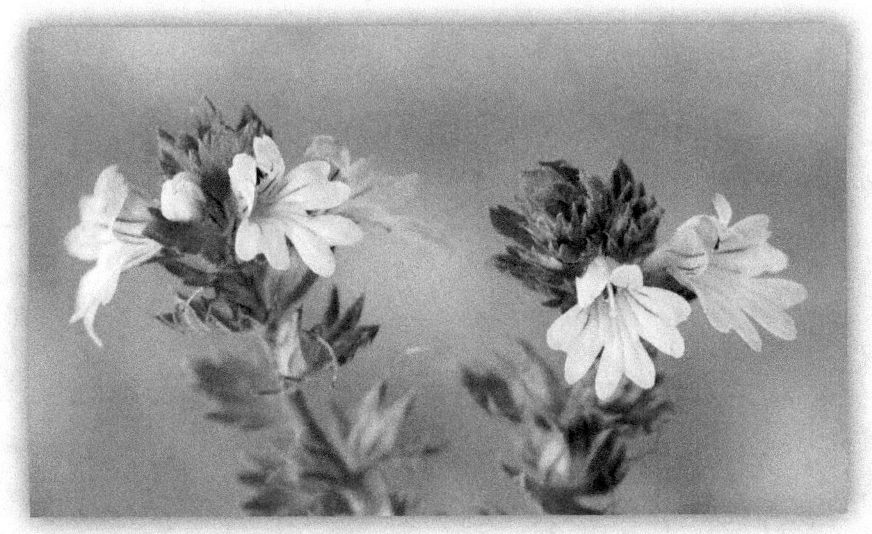

Eyebright is a perennial plant. It can be found all around the world. Eyebrights grow up to 8 inches tall and have small daisy-type flowers that bloom in late spring. It can be found in fields, woods, and meadows.

The benefit of Eyebright is that it can help clear reddened, irritated eyes. It also helps prevent conjunctivitis and infections. The flower of eyebright is used to make tea, which can help ease the pain associated with sore throats, coughs, and colds.

PREPARATION OF HERBS

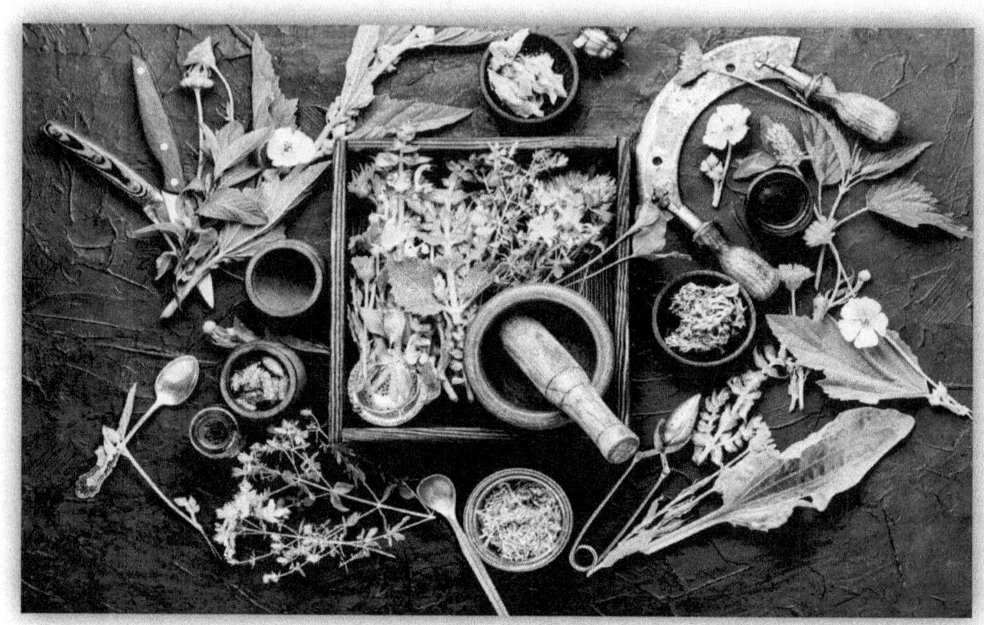

How to Prepare the Herbs

It's easier to make herbal teas with the ratio of one teaspoon to eight ounces of water for each herb. However, if making larger batches, I recommend you combine them for easier convenience on prepping and storage.

For easier batch preparation, prepping, and storage, I recommend preparing herbs in batches of mixtures. Again, this will depend on how the state of health/illness and what minerals are most important for you. You can combine similar herbs with similar functions into a batch. Like our healer, Dr. Sebi would say, "if you want calcium, you know where to go to (sea moss), if you want Iron, you go to Burdock, and if

you want a mix of both Iron and Fluorine, you go to Lily of the Valley."
In all, try not to mix more than 2 or 3 herbs together. Remember, these
herbs are electric, and it's best to preserve their organic carbon,
hydrogen, and oxygen nature as much as we can. Again, if you mix
more than that, you may not get their accurate concentrations per ml
of water, so try to limit to 3, possibly 2. For a clearer understanding,
you can try the following options:

- Mix the colon and gallbladder cleansing herbs
- Mix liver and kidney cleansing herbs
- Mix respiratory and mucus cleansing herbs
- Mix lymphatic and heavy metal cleansing herbs

Since these herbs perform a whole-body cleanse (not just colon),
including the skin, eyes, colon, liver, lymphatic system, and gallbladder,
you can decide to choose how to combine them.

For pre-purchase cleansing packages:

Please follow the recommended dosage or instructions that are
provided for that cleansing package, such as from Dr. Sebi's cell food
website. If you order the cleansing package, there are directions on
how you should consume the herbs.

For Leafy purchased herbs — For fresh Green leafy herbs:

1. Place in spring water and boil on low heat for 5 to 7 min
2. For dried leafy herbs, boil longer – 10 to 15 min

For Dried ground (or powder) herbs:

For dried ground or powder leaves or roots, mix in recommended ratios for the herb. Powder herbs are the easiest to mix in dosage proportions, so you can simply follow the package instructions.

For Chunks of Dried Root herbs:

If you're having like the chunks of the root, you can cut that up yourself.

1. Cut or break up chunks
2. Place in spring water and boil for 15 minutes
3. Let cool and serve
4. Alternatively, prepare in larger batches and place in jars to store in the refrigerator

For bulk purchase herbs:

Make herbal teas herbal teas you want to use a ratio of one teaspoon to eight ounces of water for each herb you can make larger batches of these herbs.

For capsules:

I recommend that you do research and find out what the recommended dosage is for each herbal capsule

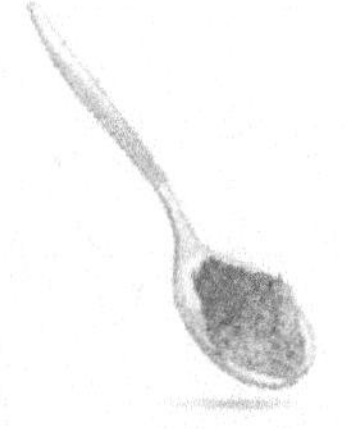 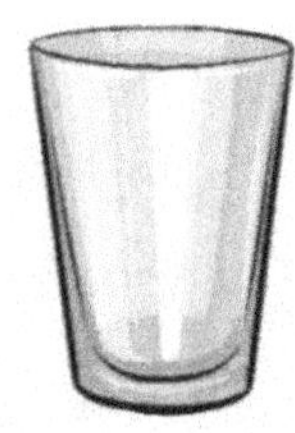

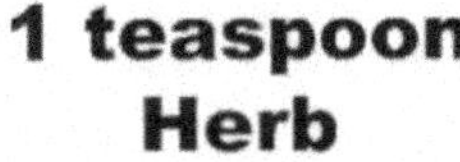

1 teaspoon Herb **+** **1 Cup (8 oz) Spring water**

How to Use These Herbs for Detoxification

If you are on medication, I recommend that you take the herbs one hour before taking your meds, as this was actually recommended by Dr. Sebi. Your cleansing herbs should not be consumed for longer than 30 days because your body may become dependent on them, and you want to start to reduce the dose during your last 3 to 5 days, depending on how long you've been taking them.

→ **Routine**

Twice a day — morning and night

→ **Daily Consistency**

Try to stay consistent in terms of timing and duration. That is, try not to skew the duration. During cleanse make it consistent. For example, for a 12-day cleanse to be taken twice daily, take them around the same time you do take them on both mornings and nights.

→ **Gradual Wean Off**

Just like medications, it is not the best to go cold-turkey when it comes to herbal detox. Towards the cleanse ends, wean off your herbs by gradually reducing the dosage and/or duration. The wean duration will depend on the length of the fast you choose. For example, for a one-month fast, I usually start weaning a week towards closure. For the standard 12 days fast, I begin weaning on day 9 or 10. You can begin to wean by reducing it from twice a day to once a day. Alternatively, simply take half the dosages each for mornings and night.

It is important you do this because you need to signal to your body to begin to prepare to start functioning on its own — without dependence on the cleansing herbs. In addition, no other way than to take it slow and do it gradually without bringing too much "shock" to the body.

What Are the Benefits of Dr. Sebi's Detoxifying Herbs?

These herbs approved by Dr. Sebi do the following:

- Provides energy for the body

- Revitalize the body

- Remove toxic waste from the body

- Multiply cells in the body

- Provide the body with irons, which is very important for the cure of the herpes virus

- Cleanses and promotes blood

THE GENERAL USES OF DR. SEBI'S HERBS TO DETOXIFY ELECTRIC BODY

Different alkaline herbs are used to detoxify different organs and locations in the body because of their different therapeutic properties in those alkaline herbs.

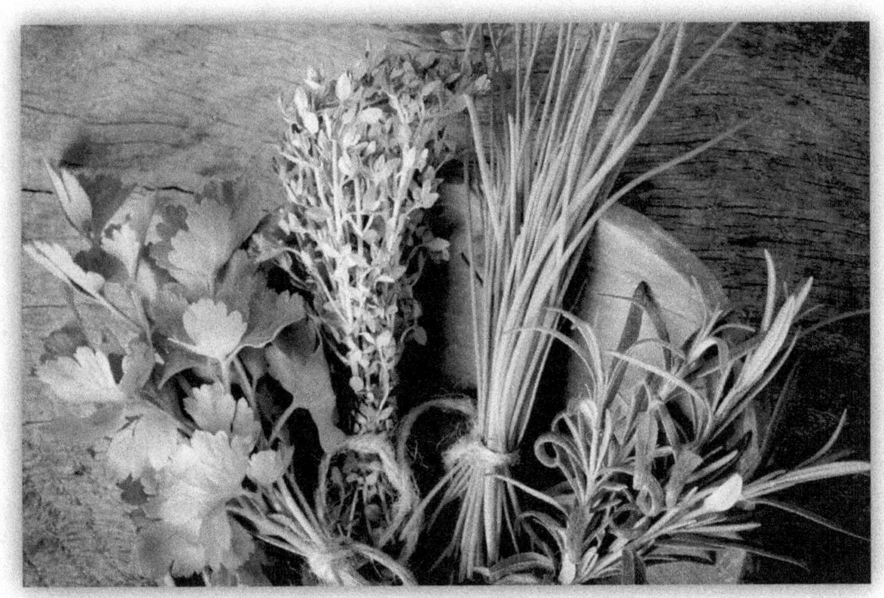

Dr. Sebi's Detox for Alimentary and Digestive Organs

In a situation of cleansing and detoxifying digestive channels and alimentary canal, Dr. Sebi used the following alkaline herbs during his lifetime.

- Rhubarb Herb

- Cascara Sagrada Herb

- Haritaki Fruit or Triphala Herb

Rhubarb Herb

The root of Rhubarb is inevitable in the preparation of medicinal detox to purify the colon and digestive canal. Rhubarb has antibacterial and anti-inflammatory properties to get rid of bacteria and reverses any existing inflammation caused by the bacteria or deposited toxins (poisons).

Cascara Sagrada Herb

This is another wonderful muscular enhancing plant the increases the auto-descending movement of the alimentary canal that prevents regurgitation (flowing back) of the ingested medicinal herbs or diets.

Cascara also improves the effective release of digestive enzymes that produce in the stomach, liver, and pancreas.

Triphala Herb

You may Triphala as powder of the fruit of Haritaki that has a laxative property, which helps the rapid digestion of food without fiber and gives room for easy free movement of bowel without any difficulty in defecating that is excretion feces.

The laxative effect helps the cleansing of the blood and bowel and the removal of coliforms (i.e. germ residing in the colon) that may be releasing abnormal gas due to their various microbial activities performing in the lumen/cavity of the intestine (colon).

Herbal Recipes

- 1teaspoon of Rhubarb Powder
- 1teaspoon of Cascara Sagrada Powder
- 1teaspoon of Triphala/Haritaki Fruit Powder

How to Make the Herbs Ready for Use

1. Separately get the herbs.
2. Carefully rinse them separately.
3. Cut the big plant into pieces.
4. Dry them under sunlight or use a hot-air oven.
5. Separately pulverize them into a powdered form by grinding.
6. From their separate container take one teaspoon of each herb and pour them inside a put.
7. Add two tumblers of water.
8. At the boiling stage, allow it to boil for extra 7minutes.
9. Filter out the particles.
10. Drink it before you go to bed for 30 days without missing a day.

Efficacious Detox for Skin, Senses, Bones, Muscles, Nerves, and Immune System

The alkaline medicinal herbs are used to detoxify skin, muscles, senses, bones nerves, reproductive and immune systems; they are also capable of calming the body system to improve stored energy (potential), body resetting, auto-cleansing ability, antiseptics, and anti-inflammation for quick recovery.

Dr. Sebi has recommended herbs be:

- Blue Vervain Herb

- Linden or Tila Herb

- Santa Maria Herb (Pericon, Mexican Marigold or Yerbanis).

- Lavender Herb

Blue Vervain Herbs

The herb is an amazing nerve relaxing natural stimulant with anti-anxiety and anti-inflammatory. It calms body nerves; improves natural immunity and controls heart function.

Linden or Tila Herb

The herb aids instant relief of red painful swollen tissues, prevents convulsion, and headache, removes depression, relaxes nerves, and muscular tissues.

Santa Maria Herb

This herb is a widely used anti-inflammatory alkaline herb; also has micronutrient components that can completely remove the causes of depression and induces calming property to relax the muscle and nervous system.

Lavender Herbs

It is antispasmodic, calming, has a sedative function and fights infections. In fact it has detoxifying properties and strong anti-septic, bactericidal and anti-inflammatory properties.

Herbal Recipes

- ½ teaspoonful of Blue Vervain Powder

- ½ teaspoonful of Linden or Tila Powder

- ½ teaspoonful of Santa Maria Powder

How to Make the Herbs Ready for Use:

1. Separately get the herbs.

2. Carefully rinse them separately.

3. Cut the big plant into pieces.

4. Dry them under sunlight or use a hot-air oven.

5. Separately pulverize them into a powdered form by grinding.

6. From their separate container take half a teaspoon of each herb and pour them inside a put.

7. Add two tumblers of water.

8. At the boiling stage, allow it to boil for extra 7minutes.

9. Filter out the particles.

10. Prepare the tea extract three times daily.

11. Drink the tea extract after the meal in the morning, afternoon, and at night before bed continually for 20 to 30 days.

Detox for Liver, Kidney, Heart, Lungs, and Blood Tissues

The selection of these herbs for the detoxification and cleansing of the essential organs in the electric body was formulated carefully and skillfully by Dr. Sebi.

As a competent herbal practitioner, he was able to understand all the various associated medicinal and nutritional properties of all the recommended herbs.

The alkaline herbs include:
- Burdock Herb
- Sarsaparilla Herb
- Bladderwrack Herb
- Nettle Herb
- Yellow Duck Herb
- Elderberry Herb

Burdock Herb

The root part of the Burdock contains a huge proportion of constituents neutralizing toxins that are capable of detoxifying the essential organs and save them from further deterioration.

Sarsaparilla Herb

The root region of the plant contains more properties of antibiotics to get rid of bacteria out of the body and anti-inflammation to arrest any inflammation in the organs and their environment.

Bladderwrack Herb

The powdered form of Bladderwrack is loaded with several micronutrients and natural vitamins that fortify the important organs and resuscitate/restore the reduced essential micronutrients.

Nettle Herb

The root of the Nettle herb contains a laden anti-toxic property that enhances cardiovascular strength, healthy function, and the neutralization of toxins in the heart, liver, lung, kidney, and blood tissues.

Yellow Duck Herb

The root of Yellow Duck is used to produce constituents neutralizing toxins and anti-inflammatory properties to detox all the organs and blood tissues.

Elderberry Herb

The flower of Elderberry is used to produce the appropriate amount of anti-toxic property for the organs detox, cleansing, and fortification.

Herbal Recipes:

- ½ teaspoon of Burdock Root Powder

- ½ teaspoon of Sarsaparilla Root Powder

- ½ teaspoon of Bladderwrack Root Powder

- ½ teaspoon of Nettle Root Powder

- ½ teaspoon of Yellow Duck Root Powder

- ½ teaspoon of Elderberry Flower Powder

How to Make the Herbs Ready for Use:

1. Separately get the herbs
2. Carefully rinse them separately.
3. Cut the big plant into pieces.
4. Dry them under sunlight or use a hot-air oven.
5. Separately pulverize them into a powdered form by grinding.

6. From their separate container take half a teaspoon of each herb and pour them inside a put.

7. Add three to four tumblers of water.

8. At the boiling stage, allow it to boil for extra 7minutes.

9. Filter out the particles.

10. Divide the whole boiled herbal extract into two equal parts.

11. Drink half before the meal in the morning and the remaining half after the meal at night before you step on the bed for 30 days without missing a day.

Dr. Sebi's Body Fortifier

The herbs for the body vitamins and essential micronutrients fortification were consciously composed by Dr. Sebi to restore every removed vital nutrient during the growth of germs, and cleansing of the body that involve the killing of germs and flushing out of some impurities.

These alkaline herbs are awesome to adequately provide the cellular strength, and power to fast track rapid growth of the cells, production of the efficient resistance against stress, infection, and hormonal imbalance.

These herbs are classified as the revitalization to revitalize the sufferers and build body their immunity.

Dr. Sebi's approve alkaline herbs to revitalize and boost natural body essential micronutrients for great sustainable healthy living are:

- Valerian Herb

- Chaparral Herb

- Stinging Nettle Herb

- Hombre Grande Herb

- Yerba Santa Herb

Valerian Herb

The extract of the root of the herb enhances the nerves and muscle calmness when it moves blood tissue containing oxygen to the brain circulation. The herb also improves the activation of blood capillaries to be more active in conveying blood tissue to terminal joints and muscles in the body.

Chaparral Herb

The herb is a fantastic herb that improves the easy flow and function of the lungs, which supercharges the healthy inhalation and exhalation of respiratory activities; more so, it rapidly arrests muscular bone joints' inflammation.

Stinging Nettle Herb

The leaves of this herb are the appropriate part that is adequately sufficient to cleanse all organs and produce long-lasting strength and vitality. The regular use of the herb ensures longevity and prevents tiredness.

Hombre Grande Herb

The herb improves natural immunity and resistance against germ-like fungi from infecting vital organs of the electric body. It enhances the function of the digestive enzymes that aid the easy digestion of any ingested food and prevent constipation.

Yerba Santa Herb

The leaves of the herb are medicinally recommended to control sugar concentration in the bloodstream and prevent or arrest joints, bones, muscle, and kidney inflammation.

Herbal Recipes

½ teaspoon Valerian Powder

½ teaspoon Chaparral Powder

½ teaspoon Nettle (Stinging) Powder

½ teaspoon Hombre Grande Power

½ teaspoon Yerba Santa Power

How to Make the Herbs Ready for Use

1. Separately get the herbs.
2. Carefully rinse them separately.
3. Cut the big plant into pieces.
4. Dry them under sunlight or use a hot-air oven.
5. Separately pulverize them into a powdered form by grinding.
6. From their separate container take half a teaspoon of each herb and pour them inside a pot.
7. Add two tumblers of water.
8. At the boiling stage, allow it to boil for extra 7minutes.
9. Filter out the particles.
10. Drink the completely boiled herbal extract after a meal in the morning and repeat the preparation at night before your bedtime.

DR. SEBI SUPPLEMENTS

Dr Sebi has created and produced a series mi mix of plants that purify, strengthen and energize the body, both as supplements and for the hygiene of the body.

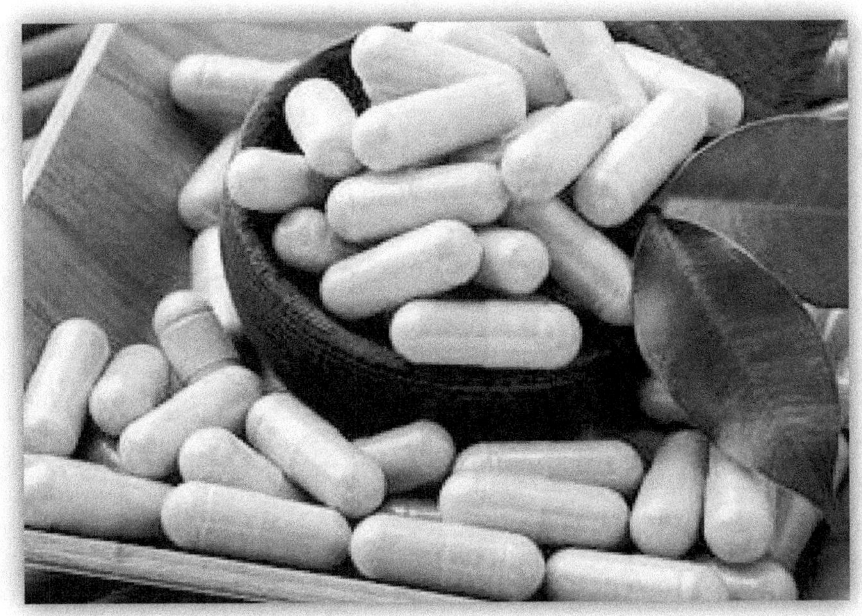

Viento

Viento is working as a revitalization, cleanser, and energizer. It contains chaparral, which is considered a powerful antioxidant. Native Americans have used Chaparral for centuries to help treat issues like pain caused by arthritis, snakebites, chickenpox, and respiratory illnesses. Since chaparral has so many antioxidants, it can help with overall wellbeing, weight loss, improve immunity, cleanse the blood, and improve the health of the liver. It has commonly been used to help treat respiratory tract problems and digestive issues like gas and cramps. The herbs found in viento include:

- Hombre Grande *(improves digestive system, intestines, immune system)*

- Hierba del Sapo *(the plant is mainly known for its aperitif, diuretic and liver depurative properties)*

- Valeriana *(anti-stress and calming)*

- Bladderwrack *(fortifying, antioxidant)*

- Chaparral *(purifying)*

Testo

Testo is a natural testosterone booster. In fact, it is the only all-natural testosterone booster in the world. It is designed specifically to target male hormonal imbalance and serves to restore the natural balance that the body's testosterone needs. It contains sarsaparilla and Irish Sea moss, among other nutritious herbs. Restore testosterone to a healthy level.

Benefits:

- Balances male hormones
- Boosts libido
- Encourages healthy blood flow
- Supports a healthy prostate

Iron Plus

Iron plus is meant to help purify the entire body. It contains chaparral, which, as we have talked about, is a powerful antioxidant. Iron plus also contains:

- Bugleweed
- Palo guaco
- Hombre Grande
- Blue vervain
- Chaparral
- Elderberry

Green Food

This multi-mineral supplement of herbs from Africa and offers chlorophyll-rich food that nourished the body. It contains ortiga, which is well known as an anti-inflammatory. It can also help with gout, rheumatism, influenza, hemorrhage, cardiovascular system, locomotor system disorders, gastrointestinal tract disorders, urinary tract infections, and kidney disorders. It is also great at helping poor circulation and purifying the blood. Ortiga has also been used to help the symptoms of hay fever. Green food contains:

- Bladderwrack
- Nopal
- Tila
- Nettle

Bromide Plus Powder/Bromide Plus Capsules

This is meant to help your thyroid gland and bones. It is great for people who suffer from dysentery, respiratory issues, pulmonary illnesses, and bad breath. It is a natural diuretic, improves the digestive system, regulates the bowels, and suppresses the appetite. It contains bladderwrack, which is a seaweed that lives in the Baltic Sea, Atlantic Ocean, and the Pacific Ocean. It is one of the original sources of iodine. It is full of mannitol, alginic, potassium, bromine, and beta-carotene. It contains bladderwrack and Irish Sea moss.

You can also get the bromide plus in capsule form if you would prefer not to drink it as a tea. They both do the same thing for your body and contain the exact same ingredients. They are simply taken in different ways.

Bio Ferro Tonic/Bio Ferro Capsules

Bio Ferro contains the right ingredients to purify and nourish the blood. It contains yellow dock root, which is an herb that acts as a digestive bitter to help improve digestion. It is a detoxifier and blood purifier and especially helps the liver. Yellow dock root also helps the digestion of fats and stimulates bile production. It can also help the intestinal track with bowel movements, and get rid of waste lingering It will also increase urination.

Bio Ferro contains:

- Cocolmeca

- Yellow dock root

- Burdock root

- Chaparral

- Elderberry

The bio ferro capsules work the same way as the tonic. They have slightly different ingredients even though they do the same thing.

The capsules contain:

- Yellow dock root
- Nopal
- Nettle
- Burdock root
- Chaparral

Banju

The banjo tonic is made from powerful ingredients to make a tonic that helps to stimulate the central nervous system and brain. It contains:

- Bugleweed

- Valerian root

- Burdock root

- Blue vervain

- Elderberry

Body Care

Uterine Oil and Wash

As you can guess by the name, this is meant for women. This helps to cleanse and restore the flora and fauna of the vagina. The red clover in the wash acts as a blood purifier, improves circulation, and acts as an expectorant. It also contains isoflavones and flavonoids, which help to produce estrogen. Red clover is great at treating conditions that are associated with menopause. The ingredients in the wash include:

- Red clover
- Sage
- Arnica
- Lupulo

Tooth Powder

You can use this natural powder as a toothpaste that will help stop gum disease and tooth decay. It contains Encino and myrrh gum powder.

Testo

This is a product just for men. This works as a natural testosterone booster and male enhancer. The formulation combines the right herbs to make a powerful synergy that increases your testosterone back to its correct levels. It helps to support the male hormonal balance. It also improves your stamina, endurance, and strength. It also helps your prostate health, healthy blood flow to the penis, and improves sexual desire. It contains:

- Irish sea moss
- Capadulla
- Locust bark
- Yohimbi
- Sarsaparilla

Hair Food Oil

This is meant to nourish the scalp and hair. It is gentle on the skin so that it can be used every day. It helps stimulate hair growth. It contains:

- French vanilla
- Coconut oil
- Batana
- Olive oil

Eyewash

This product naturally cleanses and nourishes the eye. It contains the only eyebright, which is commonly used to help treat many different eye diseases. It can also help to reduce the inflammation in the eye caused by conjunctivitis and blepharitis.

Eva Salve

This salve is meant to tone and nourish the skin. The unique combination of ingredients in Eva Salve provides natural minerals the skin needs as potassium phosphate, fluorine, and calcium, which your skin needs to maintain elasticity. It also contains sage, which is a powerful antioxidant that helps to fight off free radical damage.

Eva salve contains:

- Manzo
- Eucalyptus
- Sage
- Arnica
- Olive oil
- Lily of the valley
- Nopal
- Shea butter

Estro

This one is for women and is a natural anti-inflammatory and antioxidant. It contains damiana, which has 22 different flavonoids. For centuries, damiana has been used as an aphrodisiac. It can also help to increase and maintain healthy levels of physical and mental stamina. Estro contains:

- Irish sea moss
- Sarsaparilla
- Damiana
- Hydrangea

Herbal Teas

Stomach Relief Tea

This tea contains only cuachalalate, which is an herb used in Central America that helps provide relief for kidney sickness, gastric ulcers, stomach cancer, and other gastric and stomach pain. This can also help people find relief from kidney and urinary discomfort, minor wounds, and mouth diseases.

Stress Relief Tea

This is simply a chamomile tea that helps to provide a gentle sleeping and relaxation aid. Chamomile works as a mild sedative and can help to improve a person's mood. It relaxes tense muscles and reduces irritability. It can also help with many stomach troubles, including IBS. It also works as an antioxidant, anti-bacterial, and anti-inflammatory.

Immune Support Tea

This tea provides you with the antioxidant benefits of elderberry. Elderberries are great at reducing the swelling in the mucous membranes. It can also help relieve nasal congestions, and act as an anti-carcinogen and antiviral. It boosts the immune system. Elderberry can also help with any respiratory issues, viral and bacterial infections, flu, colds, coughs, sore throats, improve vision, and lower cholesterol.

Energy Booster Tea

This tea is meant to help boost your energy levels. It can also help to increase your iron levels, which will help to carry more oxygen throughout your body. It contains muicle, which is detoxifying and an antioxidant, and it acts as a blood purifier.

Cold and Cough Tea

This tea contains gordolobo, which provides you with the relief of mullein flowers that help to ease mucus associated with the flu or cold. Since it helps to reduce phlegm, it will also relieve coughing. It can also be helpful in treating intestinal disorders, sore throat, fever, pneumonia, laryngitis, and bronchitis.

Blood Pressure Balance Tea

This tea is made from flor de manita, which helps to regular high or low blood pressure. These flowers have been used for centuries to help heart irregularities and abdominal pain. Regularly consuming this tea could help to lower your cholesterol levels and improve your cardiovascular health.

All of these supplements serve a purpose for your body and helps to improve your overall health. You get the most benefit when you combine the supplements with the Dr. Sebi diet.

DR. SEBI ALKALINE DIET TIPS FOR SUCCESSFULLY FOLLOWING THE PROGRAM

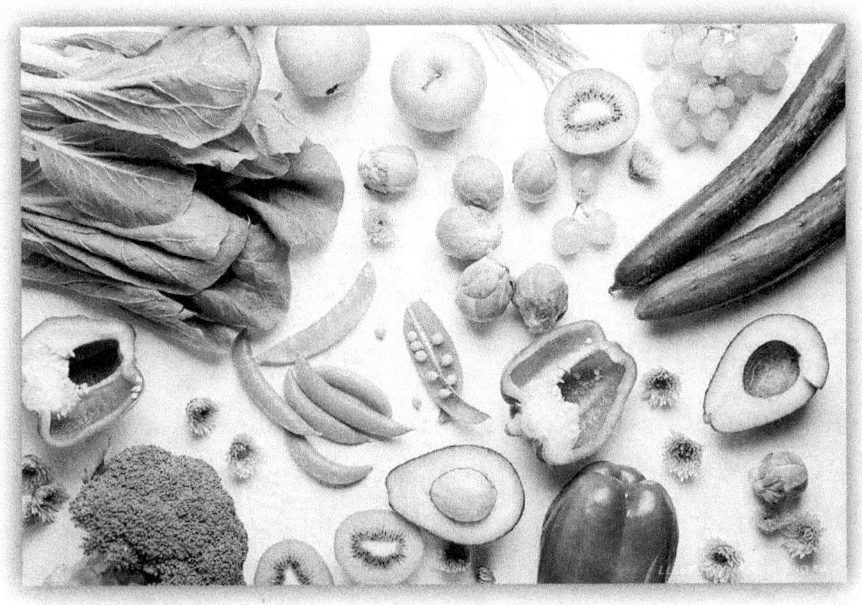

It is worth the effort all the way, all the way to that extra step to get to a healthy lifestyle, and the tool that can lead to the achievement of that goal is exactly the anti-inflammatory alkaline diet. The alkaline diet relies on the fact that by consuming foods such as fruits, vegetables, roots, and legumes, a beneficial amount of alkaline substances such as minerals: calcium, magnesium, iron, zinc, copper... minerals that strengthen the body. These take the place of harmful substances, such as waste and toxins, which are transported away from the body through the process of detoxification and purification. All of this leads to a rebirth of the vitality of our cells and mitochondria, and all our receptors finally "clean" can do their job in the body, improving all of our performance.

Some actions that can help the unfolding of this process and the success of the alkaline diet. Here are ten methods for the successful implementation of the alkaline diet.

1 -Drink water

Water is perhaps the most significant (after oxygen) resource for our body. As the water content influences, the chemistry of the body, hydration in the body is very important. To maintain the body well hydrated (filtered to cleaned), drink about 8-10 glasses of water.

2 -Stop acidic beverages like tea, coffee or soda

Our body also seeks to control the content of acid and alkali. In carbonated beverages, there is such a content of acidifying substances, that our body has to really struggle to reset the ph of the fluids inside, and many times it can't do it on its own. We need to help it by eliminating these harmful drinks!

3 - Breathe

Oxygen is the reason our body functions, and if you provide the body with ample oxygen, it can reach all the parts of our body, down to the most hidden sites to make them work better. The metabolism, the intestines, the muscles, the blood benefit so much. Sit back and enjoy deep breathing for two to five minutes. And try to do it several times a day.

4 - Avoid food with preservatives and food colors

Our body has not been conditioned to consume these chemicals, and they are then absorbed or stored as fat by the body and do not affect the liver. Acids are formed by chemicals so that the body neutralizes them either by producing cholesterol or by blanching iron from the RBCs (leading to anemia), or by removing calcium from the bones (osteoporosis).

5 - Stop artificial sweeteners

These sweeteners are potentially toxic to the body and also appear to be high in trans fats. Saccharin, the main ingredient in sweeteners, is proven to cause cancer as well. Therefore, it is best to stay away from these substances. We can recreate the sweet taste with erythritol or stevia, but it is better to gradually disabuse yourself of the addictive sweetness. After a short period of time you will no longer feel the need for it.

6 - Exercise

The exercise can also balance the alkaline element with the acidic element. Without exaggerating, to avoid that sport becomes a cause of hyper production of lactic acid. A healthy movement, even half an hour of brisk walking a day, has enormous beneficial effects on the oxygenation of muscles, bones, intestines, cardiovascular system, and is a mood enhancer. It helps to detoxify quickly and get rid of food addictions.

7 - Satiate your cravings by eating fruits, or soaked nuts for a snack

Sometimes we mistake thirst for hunger, or the need for minerals for a craving for junk food. In this case it is a good idea to bite into a fruit or nuts (previously soaked in water and lemon or apple cider vinegar, to make them more assimilable). Drinking a glass of water first is always the best choice.

8 -Eat the right food blend

When digested, carbohydrate fats and proteins require a special environment. Eating everything at once makes it very difficult to digest and assimilate, and makes you gain weight. Properly evaluate and match food composition to create the optimal mix of all nutrients in each meal.

9 - Green powders may be used as replacements for food

This helps to boost the body's alkaline consistency. Replacing a meal with herbs, gives a beneficial break to the digestive organs and liver, and at the same time purifies the body by alkalizing it.

10 - Even when under pressures, sleep well, stay calm and composed

Trying to bypass a discomfort or problem by staying calm and centered also has beneficial effects on our digestion Our mind has control over the digestive system, and you can only know that it functions properly when in a calm, centered state. Relax, then, also using breathing exercises, to detach yourself from the problems around you.

Alkaline Diet Plans

Many people nowadays find that choosing alkaline food plans is the most attractive solution to get back to health, in all aspects. As we can see, some people who have illnesses such as arthritis and cysts and people who have been obese and weak have been cured by this type of diet. Sickness is the greatest obstacle facing our lives. He/she may not do things if a person doesn't feel well, he/she might want to do it. He/she may not be able to do important things, so he/she turns to an unhealthy lifestyle. The pH equilibrium must be maintained to function properly, and the normal pH of the body must be 7,365. Our body would be alkaline rather than acidic. In this way, our body becomes alkaline and gets rid of excess acids.

By opting for alkaline diet plans, we can think of achieving:

Have the best understanding of what alkaline diet is

What the alkaline diet means is very fascinating to understand. We should note that an alkaline diet primarily consists of fresh fruits and vegetables that contain alkaline residues once metabolized in our bodies. Meat, like beef, pork, and other refined foods, is not derived from alkaline food and must therefore be eaten in limited quantities.

Plan for your meals ahead of time ahead

Preliminary meal planning is a safe way to completely value and maintain effective eating habits. It is important that the foods that you need to prioritize be listed. Although it will take some time to do so, it will be helpful as you have sufficient opportunity to reflect and write down items that can contribute to a healthier lifestyle and improved consumption.

Eat plenty of fruits and vegetables

Since alkaline foods are primarily fruits and vegetables, it is possible to eat more. These foods have negatively charged components that, when taken in by our bodies, neutralize the acids that are charged positively. Although there are some more acidic fruits and vegetables that are not recommended to be eaten in large amounts, you can choose the right alkaline vegetables.

Know P.H. balance's value

If we recognize the importance of maintaining a pH balance, we can be cautious about the types of food we consume . The fluids in our body must maintain a healthy degree of pH so that our cells continue to function properly. It does not mean, however, that we do ultimately not consume acidic foods. 75-80% of alkaline and 20-25% of acid products must be ingested to achieve a balance. It doesn't take so much time to change your life, but with the right understanding, you can make significant changes in your lifestyle. With alkaline diet plans, we just need a balanced eating schedule, then the rest...it's done from our body.

Tips for the Grocery Store

We will look at how to approach the grocery store. When you are entering the grocery store, you must do a few different things to prepare yourself, especially when beginning a new diet, as it will be challenging for you to enter the grocery store when you are having cravings and temptations while you adjust to your new diet plan. The following tips will guide you through your first number of grocery shopping experiences while you navigate this new diet.

Enter with a-List

The first thing to keep in mind when grocery shopping for a new diet is to enter with a list. By doing this, you will give yourself a guide, which will prevent you from picking up whatever you crave or whatever you feel like eating at that moment. IF you treat it like a treasure hunt, you will be able to cross things off of the list one at a time without venturing to the parts of the grocery store that you do not need to go in, and that will simply prove to be a challenge for you to avoid.

Choose Vegetables and Other Foods That You Like

Since the only things that you need to stick to are plant-based and low-carbohydrate foods and meals, you can allow yourself some room for creativity within your shopping experience. If you prefer broccoli to tomatoes, buy broccoli and find new and fun recipes to use broccoli. If you don't enjoy eggplant, you don't have to eat eggplant at all. By giving yourself some creative freedom within the parameters of your diet, you will be able to let yourself feel like you still have choice and control over what you eat, which will help you stick to the diet and avoid feelings of an uncontrolled life, which can lead you to abandon the diet quite quickly.

Ensure Your Shopping is Free of Temptations

If you are eating plant-based, you will be spending most of your time in the grocery store around the outer perimeter. This is where the whole, plant-based foods are located. By doing this, and entering with a list, as I mentioned, you will be able to avoid the middle aisles where the processed and high-carb, high-sugar foods are all kept. This will keep you away from temptations and away from foods that you will not be eating on this diet.

Don't Shop Hungry

One of the biggest things that I mention to everyone when beginning the keto diet is to shop when you are hungry. This little/big trick will get you keep going in any treat department you see. By entering the grocery store when you are full or when you have just eaten, you will be able to stick to your list and avoid falling prey to temptations.

Replacement Food for Nutrients

Let's see how to avoid stumbling into a deficiency of important nutrients, which is very often the risk one runs by following a vegan or vegetarian diet. Before starting Dr. Sebi's plant-based diet, you should make sure to to guarantee to get enough of the accompanying supplements and stock up on the following foods:

Vitamin B-12

Vitamin B-12 is an essential supplement for blood and cell health. Lack of B-12 can lead to anemia and nerve damage. B-12 is available in many animal items but not in many plant-based foods. Individuals who eat a vegan or even a vegetarian diet could consider taking a B-12 enhancement or eating foods fortified with B-12. Foods incorporate some cereals, plant-based milk, and nutritional yeast.

Iron

Individuals following Dr. Sebi's plant-based diet may have to guarantee they get enough iron in their diet, as it has lower bioavailability in plants than meat. Dr. Sebi Plant-based foods that are a decent wellspring of iron include:

- Kidney beans

- Black beans

- Soybeans

- Spinach

- Raisins

- Cashews

- Oatmeal

- Cabbage

- Tomato juice

- Dark leafy greens

Consume citrus and other vitamin C sources with plant-based wellsprings of iron to increase absorption.

Protein

Some individuals may have worries about getting enough protein from Dr. Sebi's plant-based diet. However, there is a wide variety of plant-based wellsprings of protein, including:

- Lentils

- Chickpeas

- Quinoa

- Beans, for example, kidney, pinto, or black beans

- Tofu

- mushrooms

- Nuts

- Seeds

Consuming proteins from a variety of food sources can help give all the amino acids for good health. For example, individuals could add a handful of seeds or a spoonful of hummus to tofu or beans. Remember to always soak beans, and legumes, for many hours, and cook them very long and on low flame. This allows the elimination of the anti-nutrients contained in legumes, as well as making them more bio-available and less irritating for the bowel.

Omega-3 Fatty Acids

Omega-3 fatty acids are vital as they help lessen inflammation, memory misfortune, and other eternal conditions, for example, heart disease. The two-primary omega-3 fatty acids are E.P.A. and D.H.A. Fish, seafood, and animal items, eggs are among the primary sources E.P.A. and D.H.A. White several plants-based foods, for example, walnuts, hempseed, and flaxseed contain omega-3 A.L.A., research shows that the body is moderate and wasteful at changing over A.L.A. to E.P.A. and D.H.A. Some individuals are also genetically at risk for poor absorption of A.L.A. Vegetarians show lower levels of D.H.A. and E.P.A. in blood and tissue, which may increase inflammation, memory difficulties, brain mist, and different effects. Individuals following Dr. Sebi's plant-based diet should note an omega-3 enhancement, both through attention to dietary combinations and a range of plant-based omega-3 supplements that is available for purchase on the web. It should be noted that many dietitians advise vegetarians to decrease the amount of professional inflammatory linoleic acid they consume. Soybean, corn, safflower oils, and sunflower contain linoleic acid.

THE 5 MUSTS OF FOODS

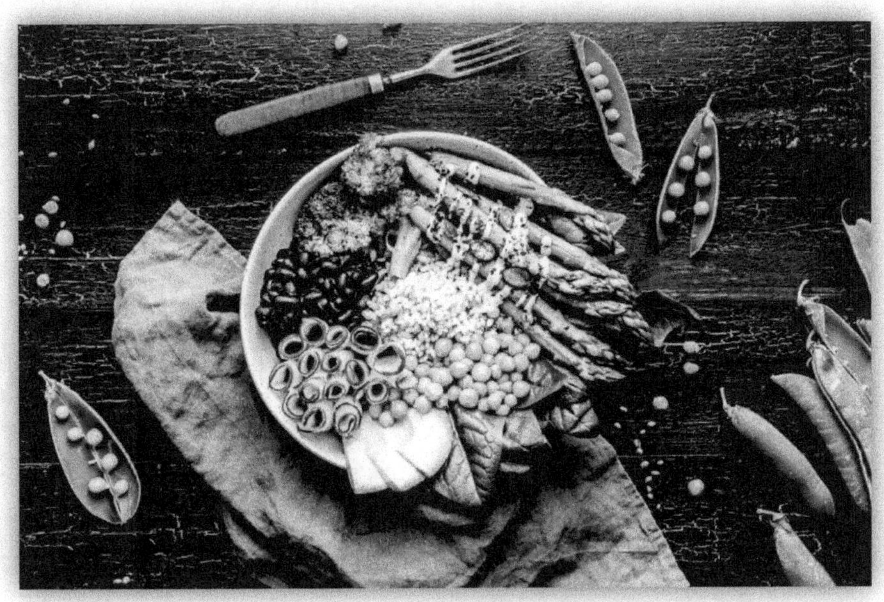

We are going to look at the five things you must do when it comes to your food. These five things simply have to do with how you prepare or store your foods, as well as things you should consume every day for a successful diet and a healthy body.

- **Cooking your food is not going to harm its electricity.**

  I wanted to get this one out of the way right off the bat. For a long time, people have been spreading the lie that cooking your food will cause it to lose its electricity. Many people live their life thinking, "raw food is better than cooked food." According to Dr. Sebi, food can't be destroyed. You can eat it raw, you can eat it cooked, you can grind it into carbon and drink it, but it is still going to be electrical. If what you are eating is real food, you are not going to be able to destroy its energy.

You can't destroy any other energy, so why would you be able to destroy the energy in food? You can change its state, but you cannot destroy its energy. There are things that people call food, but it's not real food. It is just garbage because it is full of starch, and that is already a loser in the beginning, lacking any energy. In an interview, Dr. Sebi talked about people who eat "raw foods" because it is "healthier." He shares that when he first arrived in New York, there were many "raw" people, but they were eating raw starch and they were anemic. They may have been eating "raw food," but it wasn't real natural food.

You are able to eat food in any state that you want to because it cannot be destroyed. Food is energy, and energy cannot be destroyed. Just as Dr. Sebi has said repeatedly, why would his diet have been able to cure people of leukemia and AIDS if cooked foods lost their electricity?

- **Consume plenty of alkalizing beverages every day, and it doesn't have to be just water.**

You are supposed to drink at least 1 liter of spring water every day, but you don't have to confine yourself to just plain spring water. You can get its alkalizing effects along with the benefits of other foods by mixing them into a delicious alkalizing beverage. One of the best things you can do for your body is to start every day with a glass of warm limewater.

As we all know, the body is made up of 60% water. Water helps to flush toxins out of the body, keeps you energized, and prevents dehydration. When you add lime, you are adding antioxidants. Limes are full of magnesium, calcium, vitamins A, B, C, and D, and potassium. Drinking limewater can help to promote healthier and younger-looking skin. The antioxidants found in the lime helps to strengthen collagen and the water will hydrate the skin. Limewater will also help your digestion. Limes work with your saliva to break down your food so that your stomach doesn't have as much work to do. This can help prevent constipation and acid reflux. Its vitamin C content can also help your out during the cold and flu season. The citric acid present in limes can also help to boost your metabolism, which will help you to store less fat and burn more calories.

Limewater isn't the only option you have. You can also enjoy any tea made from the approved herbs list. One of the most popular choices is ginger tea. Ginger is high in magnesium, vitamin C, and other minerals. Ginger tea can help to relieve nausea. It is a favorite among people who suffer from motion sickness when traveling. Drinking ginger tea before traveling can help prevent vomiting and nausea. If you are sick, drinking a cup of ginger tea at the first signs of nausea will help keep it at bay. Ginger tea is also able to help relieve congestion associated with a cold and allergies. Ginger tea is also able to improve your digestion. Drinking a cup of tea after you eat can help prevent bloating. It is also a great drink for people who have arthritis or other joint problems. Ginger tea can also help to relieve stress.

- Keep your pantry good stocked and your food preparation healthy, so your food is always intact and vital.

Remember all of the Tupperware your mother collected over the years. Think about holiday gatherings with food wrapped in plastic wrap and those Styrofoam take-home containers from your favorite restaurant. While those may be convenient and affordable, they aren't conducive to a healthy lifestyle. Plastic has invaded our life in every way possible simply because it is cheap, but what it does to our health and our environment is a big price to pay in the end. Most Americans only recycle 14% of their plastic packaging, so most of this stuff ends up on our streets or landfills.

Anything your food touches have a chance to leech into your food, but this happens with plastic at a much higher rate than others do. There are many various types of plastics, and substances are added to plastics to change how flexible it is, stabilize it, and shape it. BPA is one substance that is added to plastic to make polycarbonate plastics. Phthalates are another substance that is added to plastics in order to make them flexible and soft. Polycarbonate plastics are used in things like food storage containers, plastic plates, reusable water bottles, and even in the receipt, you get at the store. Metal cans also contain BPA-based liners so that the foods inside aren't able to corrode the can. Paper cups are lined with BPA as well so that your coffee doesn't leak through as quickly. Most plastic containers will have a code on the bottom. If you see a number from 3 to 7, it could have BPA.

Phthalates are found in many different products and can be harder to know if they are in certain items. They are in cosmetics, water, plastics, food, drugs, dust.. and air! Since

2008, manufacturers have removed some forms of phthalates from children's toys, and there are some countries have banned them from packaging. The best way to avoid phthalates is to look for PVC or the number 3. The Fair Packaging and Labeling Act require manufacturers to mark phthalates, but it is not required when they are used in fragrance.

While the FDA considered BPA safe and plastics are supposed to be tested and stable, it still has an effect on your health. Research has found that phthalates and BPA can mimic hormones, which can create an endocrine disruption. The endocrine system affects things from our sleep and immunity to our reproduction and growth. Even BPA-free containers aren't free from problems.

To make sure that your food stays healthy and doesn't soak up any of those bad chemicals present in plastic, it is important that you choose storage containers and prep items that are not made from plastic. Glass containers should be your best friend. Mason jars are a great option because they come in many different sizes, are inexpensive, and can be reused. You drink out of them, store salads, and soups, as well as seeds, nuts, spices, and herbs. Mason jars can also be used as lunch containers so that you don't have to use plastic baggies.

There are also other glass storage containers out there if you don't want to store everything in mason jars. You can even find some that are made from tempered glass so that they aren't easily broken.

Stainless steel is also a good option. There are many different sizes and shapes, and you can find them in bento box styles, insulates, and leak-proof. They tend to be more durable than glass containers, which is good if you have children. It is important to make sure that you buy 100% food-grade stainless steel and not aluminum. You will also want to make sure that your cutting board is not made from plastic as well, il legno potrebbe essere una buona opzione.

- **You should make your own veggie stocks and nut milk.**

  While everybody loves buying pre-made stocks and milk because of the convenience, they may not be the best option for your health. When you buy something that is pre-made, you have no idea what is in them. If you make them on your own, you will know what you are putting in them. When it comes to vegetable stock, the store-bought kind has a lot of salt in it, and it probably isn't pure sea salt. They probably used vegetables that aren't on the approved list as well. The great news is making your own vegetable stock isn't that hard. All you really need is spring water approve vegetables and some spices. Allow them to boil together for some time and you have vegetable stock. You'll also find that it tastes a lot better than the store-bought kind.

  As far as nut milk goes, it's hard to find one that fits on the approved list. Almond and cashew are the most common. Get this; almond milk doesn't even contain real almonds. One industry insider has stated that a half-gallon of almond milk has less than a handful of almonds. Most of them also contain additives. Many vegan milk products contain carrageenan, which comes from seaweed and acts as a thickener. There is a lot of interest concerning carrageenan. Some say it is a carcinogen and others say that it can cause inflammation, ulceration, and contains no nutritional benefits. If you like using nut milk, and there are Dr. Sebi recipes that call for walnut milk, you will need to make your own. Making your own nut milk isn't that hard to do, either, but also fun and gives a lot of satisfaction.

- **Buy your produce at the farmers' market when you can.**

Shopping at a local farmers' market gives you access to locally grown and fresh foods. The foods there are at the peak of the season, so they are going to be fresher and taste better. The produce has traveled thousands of miles to get to you, either. It probably doesn't contain any wax coatings or sprays. You are also face-to-face with the farmer, which gives you a chance to ask them about the product and find out how it was grown. You may also find produce at the farmers' market that isn't available at your local grocery store, and the prices might be a little more reasonable.

That said you don't always have the choice of shopping at the farmers' market. During the winter, you may not have as many options, and some farmers' markets may even close.

When it comes to shopping for foods, also **go with local first, and then go with organic**. The important thing is to make sure you are getting produce in its best possible state. Another option is to try growing fruits and veggies on your own. If you have space, and if the plants will grow where you live, growing your own produce can save you money and you will know exactly how it was grown. Without forgetting the energy aspect and the impact on well-being and good mood that you get from growing your own produce and making your own food. Well, even that I assure you is very alkalizing!

BONUS: THE SEVEN-DAY PLAN TO DETOX YOUR LIVER AND INTESTINE

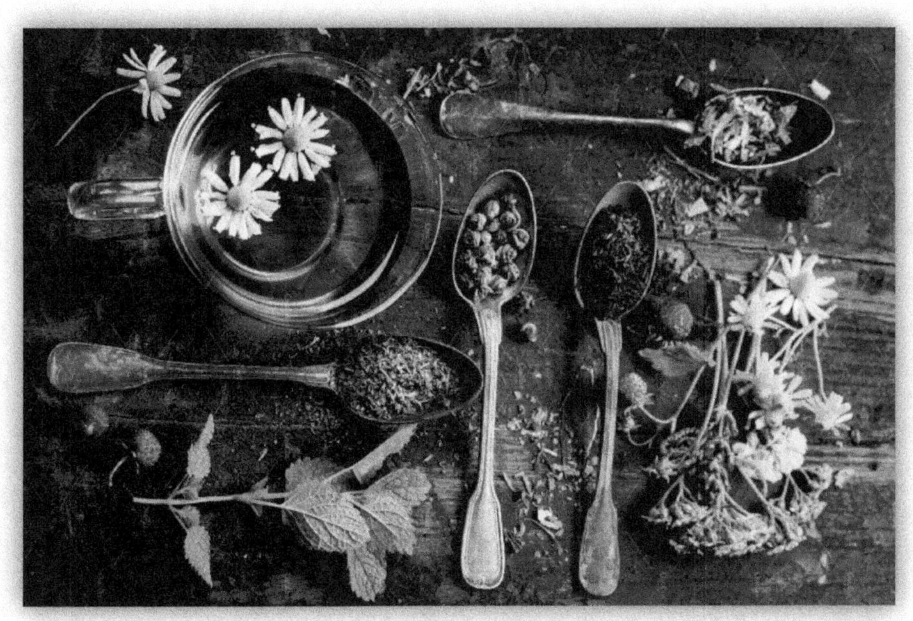

A kick start to your new alkaline life

DAY	BREAKFAST	LUNCH	DINNER	SNACK
1	Herbal Smoothie	Mushroom Risotto	Pesto Zoodles	Mucus Liver Cleansing tea
2	Peach Muffin with herbal tea	Quinoa and cherry tomato bowl	Healthy date balls	Liver-Kidney Cleansing tea
3	Triple Berry Smoothie	Mushroom coconut soup	Apple and cabbage salad	Relaxing Ashwagandha milk
4	Blueberry Smoothie	Mango and cherry tomato salad	Chickpea and Quinoa Burgers	Immune Boosting Tea
5	Raspberry, Peach, and Walnuts Smoothie	Wild rice and lentils bowl	Roasted vegetable and St. John's wort salad	Respiratory Power Boost
6	Kamut porridge with dates	"Tagliatelle" with avocado sauce	Roasted cauliflower and walnuts	Cucumber and watermelon detox smoothie
7	Blueberry Spelt Pancakes	Ratatouille and quinoa stew	Tef Grain Burger	Invigorating Sea Moss Pudding

Day 1

1. Breakfast: Herbal Smoothie

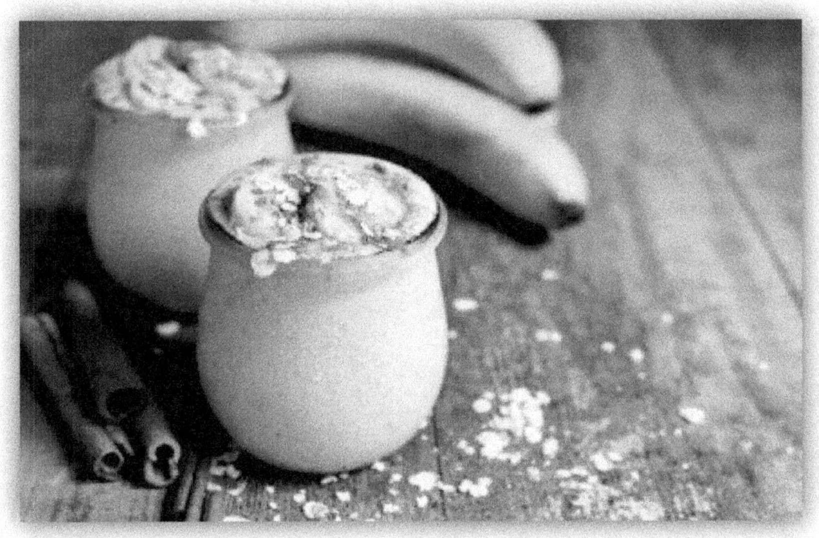

- ➤ **Preparation time:** 5 minutes
- ➤ **Servings:** 2

Ingredients:

- 2 cups Dr. Sebi's Herbal Tea
- 1 burro banana, peeled
- 1 tablespoon walnut
- 1 tablespoon agave syrup
- 1 pinch cinnamon

Directions:

1. Plug in a high-speed food processor or blender and add all the ingredients to its jar.
2. Cover the blender jar with its lid and then pulse for 40 to 60 seconds until smooth.
3. Divide the drink between two glasses and then serve.

Nutrition: Calories: 75.5, Fat: 2.1 g, Protein: 0.9 g, Carbs: 13.2 g, Fiber: 1.8 g.

2. Lunch: Mushroom Risotto

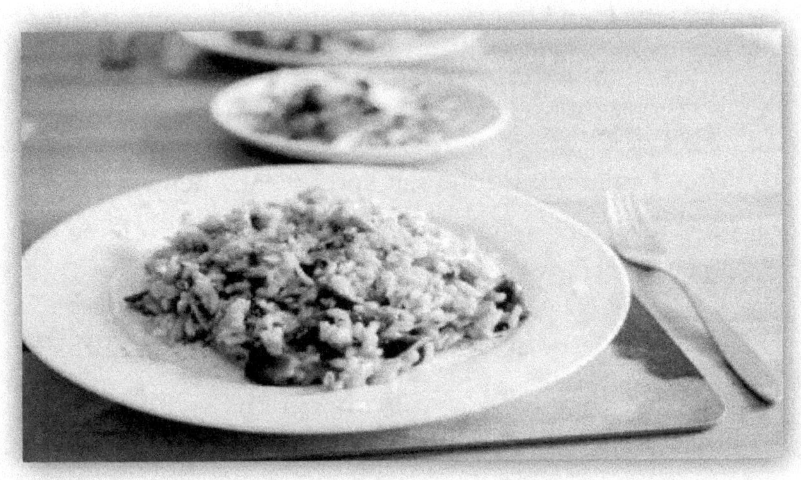

> **Preparation time:** 5 minutes
> **Cooking time:** 40 minutes
> **Servings:** 2

Ingredients:

- 4 ounces sliced mushrooms
- ¼ of an onion, chopped
- 1 cup wild rice
- 1 tablespoon grapeseed oil
- 2 cups vegetable broth, homemade
- 1/3 teaspoon salt
- ¼ teaspoon cayenne pepper

Directions:

1. Turn on the stove on medium heat, then put the olive oil in the pan and heat for a while. After that, add the onions,

mushrooms and let them cook for 4-5 minutes until they reach the right browning.

2. After the liquid has evaporated, add the rice and stir until it is mixed with the previously added ingredients and let it cook for 1 minute or more.

3. After 1 minute, add the salt and cayenne pepper, pour in the vegetable stock, reduce the heat level and leave on the heat for a while.

4. Let it cook for about 35 minutes or more, until the rice is softened and serve.Take a medium pot, place it over medium heat add oil, and when hot, add onion and mushroom and then cook for 4 to 5 minutes until mushrooms have turned golden brown and the liquid in the pan have evaporated.

5. Add rice, stir until mixed, cook for 1 minute, and then stir in salt and cayenne pepper.

6. Pour in the broth, switch heat to the low level, then cook the rice for 1 hour and 20 minutes, until rice is tender, and then serve.

Nutrition: Calories: 133, Fat: 1.3 g, Protein: 4.5 g, Carbs: 25.2 g, Fiber: 2.4 g.

3. Snack: Mucus Liver Cleansing Tea

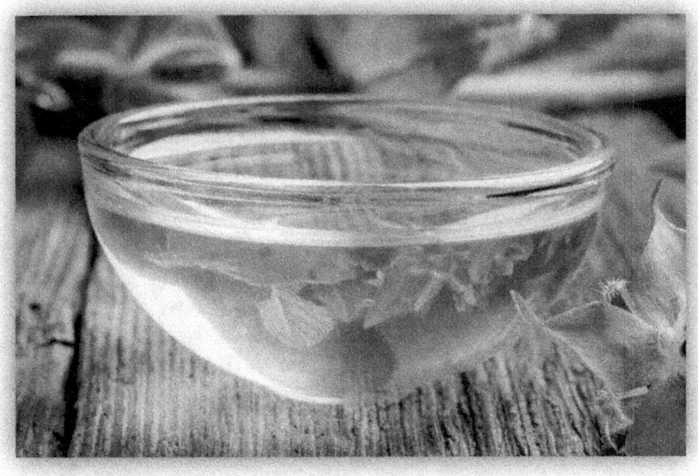

- ➢ **Preparation time:** 5 minutes
- ➢ **Cooking time: 10** minutes
- ➢ **Servings:** 1

Ingredients:

- 1 teaspoon dandelion root powder
- 1 teaspoon Prodigiosa powder
- 1 cup spring water

Directions:

1. Place dandelion and Prodigiosa powder in a tea kettle boil for 10 minutes. Remove and leave for an additional 10 minutes. Serve.

4. Dinner: Pesto Zoodles

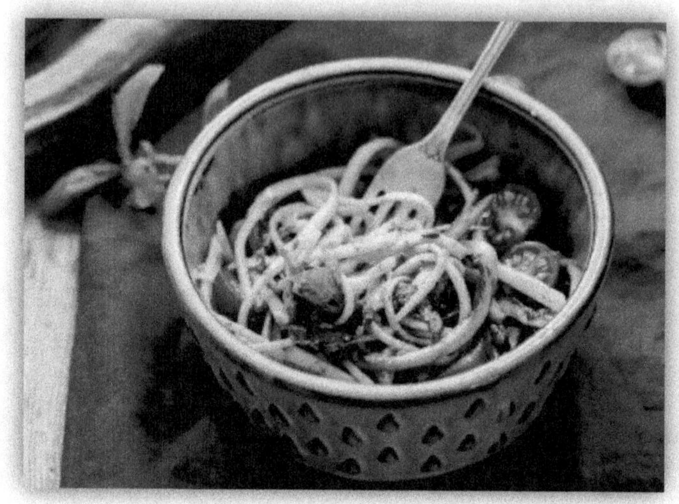

- ➤ **Preparation time:** 10 minutes
- ➤ **Cooking time:** 5 minutes
- ➤ **Servings**: 2

Ingredients:

- 2 zucchini
- 1 avocado, peeled, pitted
- ½ cup cherry tomatoes
- 2 tablespoons walnuts
- ½ of key lime, juiced
- ¼ teaspoon salt
- 1/8 teaspoon cayenne pepper
- 2 teaspoons grapeseed oil
- 2 tablespoons olive oil

- 1 tbsp grated coconu

Directions:

1. Prepare the zucchini noodles and for this, cut them into thin strips by using a vegetable peeler or use a spiralizer.
2. Then take a medium skillet pan, add oil in it and when hot, add zucchini noodles in it and then cook for 3 to 5 minutes until tender crisp.
3. Meanwhile, place the remaining ingredients in a food processor and then pulse until the creamy paste comes together.
4. When zucchini noodles have sautéed, drain and place them in a large bowl and add the blended sauce in it.
5. Add 2 tablespoons of water and then toss until well combined.
6. Garnish the zoodles with grated coconut.

Nutrition: Calories: 214, Fat: 1017.10 g, Protein: 4.8 g, Carbs: 13.2 g, Fiber: 6.1 g.

Day 2

---

5. Breakfast: Peach Muffin

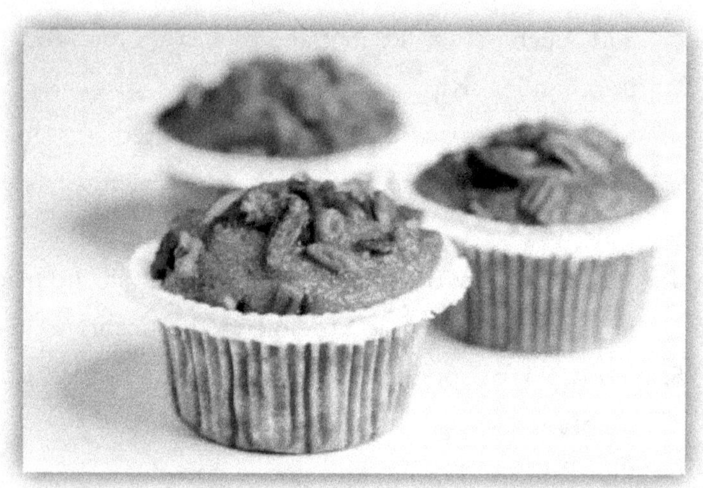

> **Preparation time:** 10 minutes
> **Cooking time:** 15 minutes
> **Servings:** 4

Ingredients:

- 2/3 cup spelt flour
- ½ of peach, chopped
- 1 teaspoon mashed burro banana
- 2/3 tablespoons chopped walnuts
- 6 ½ tablespoons walnut milk, homemade
- 1/16 teaspoon salt

- 2 2/3 tablespoon date sugar
- 2/3 tablespoon spring water, warmed
- 2/3 teaspoon key lime juice

Directions:

1. Switch on the oven, then set it to 400 °F and let it preheat.

2. Meanwhile, peel the peach, cut it in half, remove the pit, and then cut one-half of the peach into ½-inch pieces, reserving the other half of the peach for later use.

3. Take a medium bowl, pour in the milk, and then whisk in mashed banana and lime juice until well combined.

4. Take a separate medium bowl, place flour in it, add salt and date sugar, stir until mixed, whisk in milk mixture until smooth, and then fold in peached until mixed.

5. Take four silicone muffin cups, grease them with oil, fill them evenly with the prepared batter, and then sprinkle walnuts on top.

6. Bake the muffins for 10 to 15 minutes until the top is nicely golden brown and inserted toothpick into each muffin comes out clean.

7. When done, let muffins cool for 10 minutes.

Nutrition: Calories: 76.1, Fat: 3.3 g, Protein: 0.9 g, Carbs: 14.3 g, Fiber: 0.9 g

6. Lunch: Quinoa Bowl

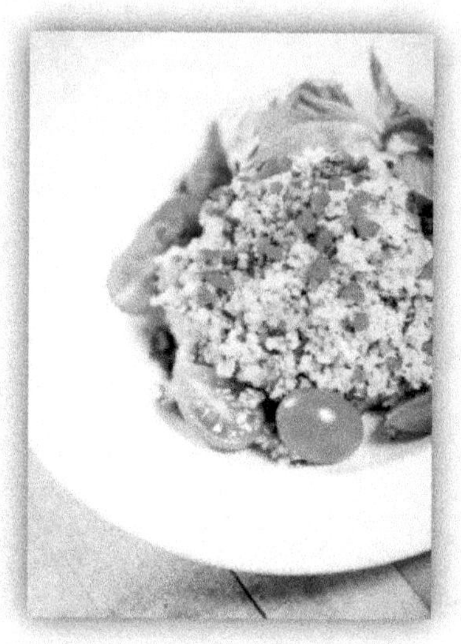

- ➤ **Preparation time:** 5 minutes
- ➤ **Cooking time:** 3 minutes
- ➤ **Servings:** 2

Ingredients:

- 1/3 cup quinoa, cooked
- ¼ cup cherry tomatoes, quartered
- ½ of green bell pepper, chopped
- 1/3 cup basil leaves
- 1 tablespoon grapeseed oil
- ¼ teaspoon salt
- 1/8 teaspoon cayenne pepper

Directions:

1. Take a skillet pan, place it over medium-high heat, add oil, and
    when hot, add cherry tomatoes and bell pepper and cook for 2
    to 3 minutes until tender-crisp.

2. Take a medium bowl, place cooked quinoa in it, add tomatoes
    and bell pepper mixture, and then add basil leaves.

3. Season with salt and cayenne pepper, stir until mixed.

Nutrition: Calories: 141, Fat: 6.2 g, Protein: 6.5 g, Carbs: 32 g, Fiber:
4.1 g.

7. Snack: Liver-Kidney Cleansing Tea

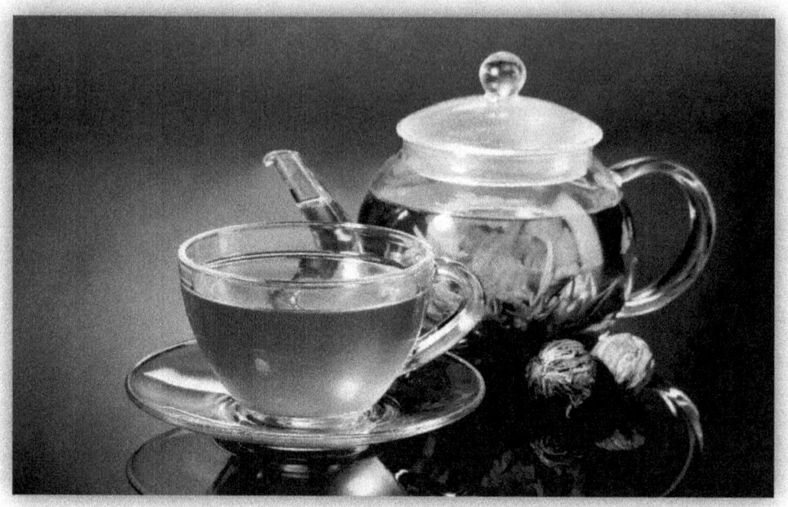

- ➢ **Preparation time:** 5 minutes
- ➢ **Cooking time:** 10 minutes
- ➢ **Servings:** 1

Ingredients:

- 1 teaspoon dandelion root powder
- 1 teaspoon burdock root powder
- 1 cup spring water

Directions:

1. Put the dandelion and burdock root powder in a tea kettle. Boil within 10 minutes, remove and leave for an additional 10 minutes. Drain and serve.

8. Lunch: Dates Healthy Balls

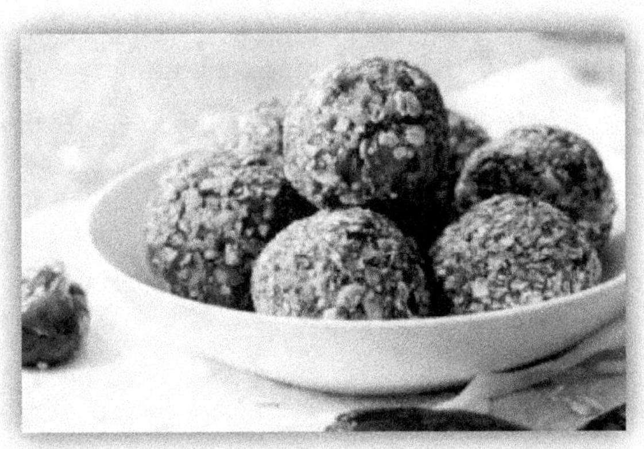

- ➢ **Preparation time:** 10 minutes
- ➢ **Cooking time:** 10 minutes
- ➢ **Servings:** 10

Ingredients:

- 1 cup of about 10 Medjool dates, pitted
- 1/2 cup raw walnuts, cashews, walnuts, almonds, pecans, etc.
- pinch of sea salt

Directions:

1. Add the dates, walnuts and salt to a food processor fitted with an S-shaped blade.

2. Process until the mixture is well combined and sticks together.

3. Form balls: Scoop the dough out of the food processor with your hands (or a cookie scoop) and form into balls with your hands. Enjoy immediately or save for later.

4. To store: Place balls in a sealed container and store in the refrigerator for 1-2 weeks or in the freezer for up to 3 months.

Nutrition: Calories: 98, Fat: 82 g, Protein: 2 g, Carbs: 10 g, Fiber: 2 g.

Day 3

9. Breakfast: Triple Berry Smoothie

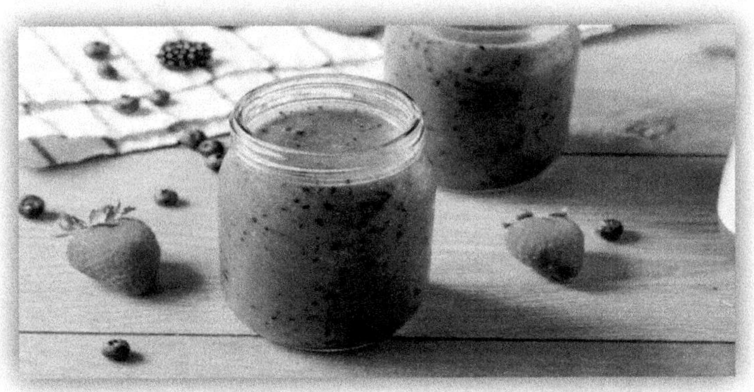

- ➢ **Preparation time:** 5 minutes
- ➢ **Servings:** 2

Ingredients:

- ½ cup strawberries
- 2 tablespoons agave syrup
- ½ cup raspberries
- 1 burro banana, peeled
- ½ cup blueberries
- 1 cup spring water

Directions:

1. Plug in a high-speed food processor or blender and add all the ingredients to its jar.
2. Cover the blender jar with its lid and then pulse for 40 to 60 seconds until smooth.
3. Divide the drink between two glasses and then serve.

10. Lunch: Breakfast: Mushroom Coconut Soup

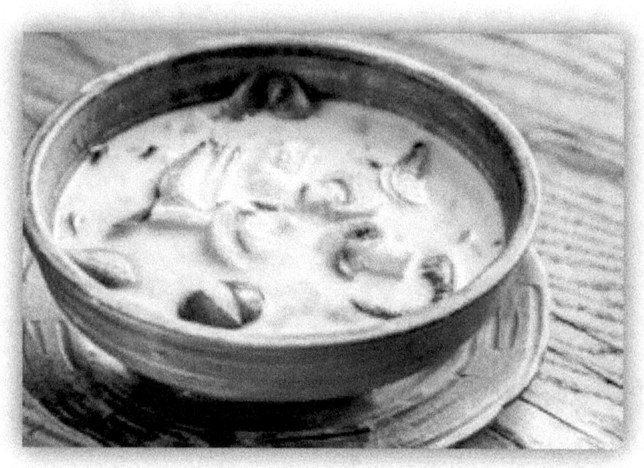

- ➢ **Preparation time:** 10 minutes
- ➢ **Cooking time:** 20 minutes
- ➢ **Servings:** 2

Ingredients:

- 2 cups baby Bella mushrooms, diced
- ½ cup diced red onions
- 1 cup vegetable broth
- 1 ½ cups soft-jelly coconut milk
- ½ teaspoon of whole sea salt
- ¼ teaspoon cayenne pepper
- 2 teaspoons grapeseed oil

Directions:

1. Take a medium saucepan, place it over medium-high heat, add oil, and when hot, add onion, mushrooms, season with salt and pepper, and then cook for 3 to 4 minutes until vegetables turn tender.
2. Then pour in milk and broth, stir until mixed and bring it to a boil.
3. Switch heat to medium-low level and then simmer the soup for 15 minutes until thickened to the desired level.
4. Serve straight away.

Nutrition: Calories: 101, Fat; 1,9 g Protein: 2 g, 18 g Carbs: 18 g, Fiber: 2 g.

11. Snack: Relaxing Ashwagandha milk

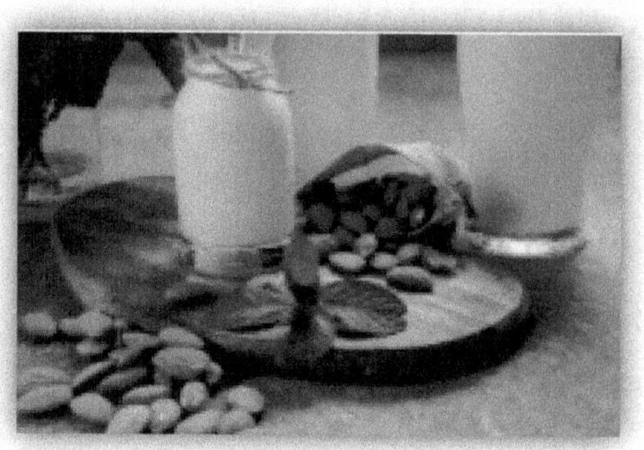

- ➢ **Preparation time:** 10 minutes
- ➢ **Cooking time:** 5 minutes
- ➢ **Servings:** 1

Ingredients:

- 1 cup of almond milk
- 1 teaspoon powder of Ashwagandha root or leaves
- 1 tablespoon almond butter
- 1 teaspoon of maple syrup

Directions:

1. Boil all ingredients for 5 minutes. Pour the milk into a preheated cup that has been run under hot water to keep the drink warm. Drain and serve.

Nutrition: Calories: 98, Carbs: 2 g, Fat: 9 g, Protein: 5 g.

12. Dinner: Apple and cabbage salad

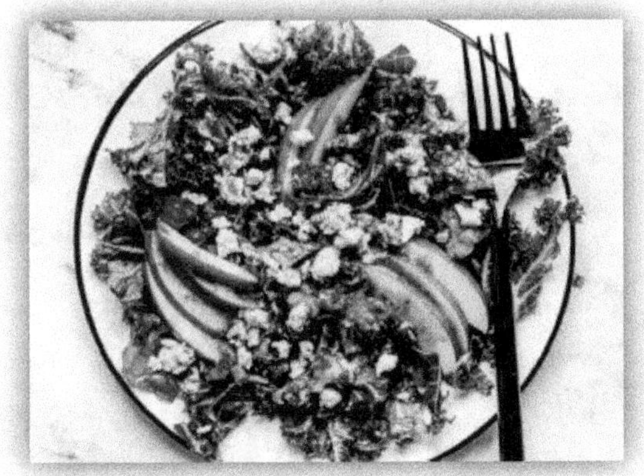

- ➢ **Preparation time:** 15 minutes
- ➢ **Cooking time:** 15 minutes
- ➢ **Servings:** 2

Ingredients:

- 3 large apples, sliced
- 6 cups fresh kale
- ¼ cup walnuts, chopped
- 2 Tbsp. olive oil
- 1 tbsp. agave nectar
- Whole grain sea salt, if needed

Directions:

1. In a salad bowl, place all ingredients: and toss to coat well with dressing.
2. Serve immediately.

Nutrition: Calories: 260, Fat: 1,3g, Protein: 5,3 g, Carbs: 38,4 g, Fiber: 6,3 g.

Day 4

13. Breakfast: Blueberry Smoothie

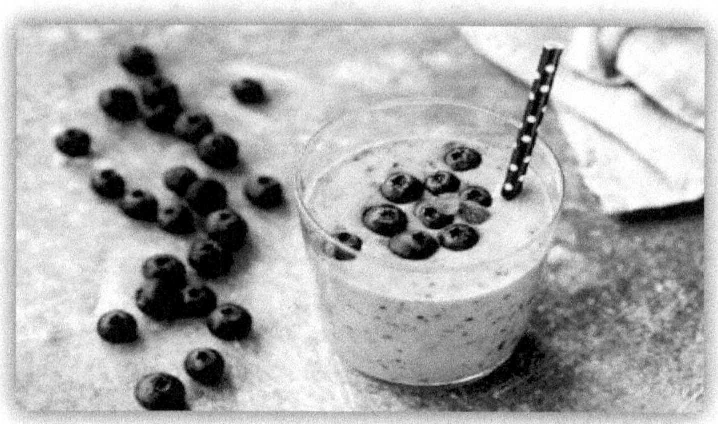

> **Preparation time:** 5 minutes
> **Servings:** 2

Ingredients:

- ½ cup blueberries
- 1 burro banana, peeled
- ¼ cup cooked quinoa
- 2 tablespoon date sugar
- 1 cup walnut milk, homemade

Directions:

1. Plug in a high-speed food processor or blender and add all the ingredients to its jar.
2. Cover the blender jar with its lid and then pulse for 40 to 60 seconds until smooth.
3. Divide the drink between two glasses and then serve.

Nutrition: Calories: 194, Fat: 5 g, Protein: 5 g, Carbs: 34 g, Fiber: 2 g.

14. Lunch: Mango and cherry tomato Salad

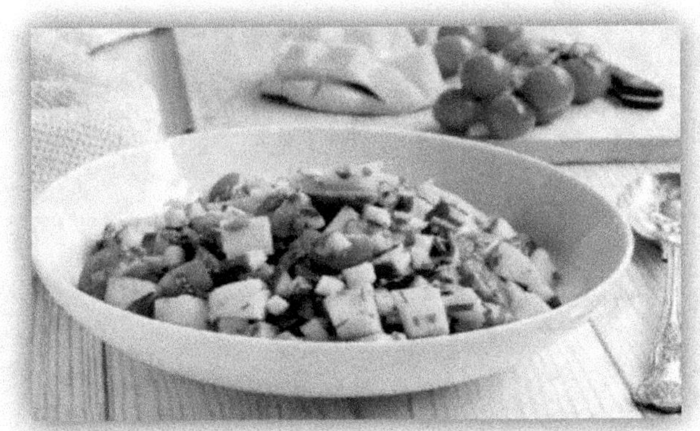

- ➢ **Preparation time:** 10 minutes
- ➢ **Servings:** 2

Ingredients:

- 1 mango, peeled, destoned, cubed
- ¼ of onion, chopped
- ½ cup cherry tomatoes halved
- ½ of cucumber, deseeded, sliced
- ½ of green bell pepper, deseeded, sliced
- 1 pinch whole sea salt
- ¼ teaspoon cayenne pepper
- ¼ of key lime, juiced

Directions:

1. Take a medium bowl, place the mango pieces in it, add onion, tomatoes, cucumber, and bell pepper, and then drizzle with lime juice.
2. Season with salt and cayenne pepper, toss until combined, and let the salad rest in the refrigerator for a minimum of 20 minutes.

Nutrition: Calories: 108, Fat: 0.5 g, Protein: 1 g, Carbs: 28.1 g, Fiber: 3.3 g.

15. Snack: Immune Boosting Tea

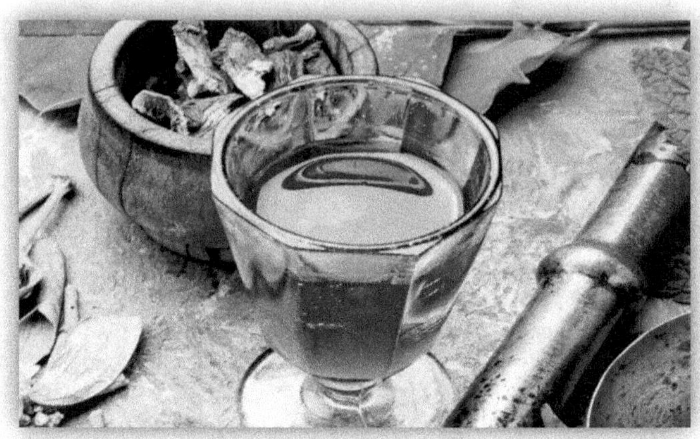

- ➤ **Preparation time:** 5 minutes
- ➤ **Cooking time:** 7 minutes
- ➤ **Servings:** 1

Ingredients:

- 1 teaspoon linden powder
- 1 cup spring water

Directions:

1. Boil linden powder in a tea kettle with spring water within 5 minutes.
2. Drain and serve.

16. Dinner: Chickpea and Quinoa Burgers

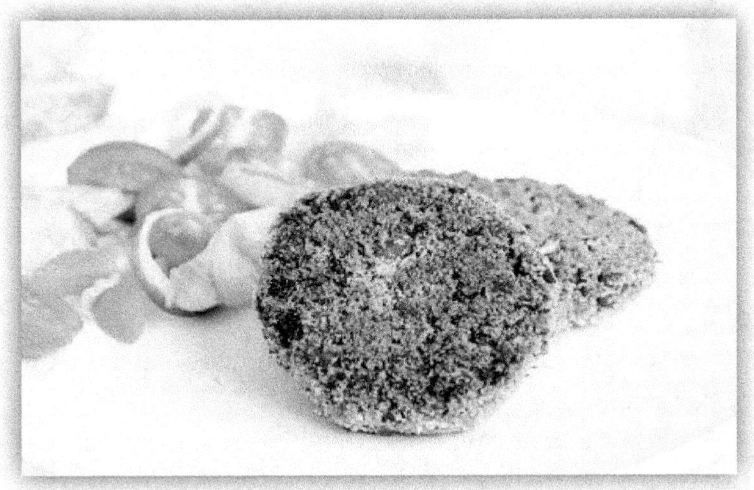

> ➤ **Preparation time:** 10 minutes
> ➤ **Cooking time:** 20 minutes
> ➤ **Servings:** 2

Ingredients:

- 2 tablespoons chopped onion
- ¾ cup chickpeas
- ¼ cup cooked quinoa
- 1 tablespoon spring water
- 1 tablespoon grapeseed oil
- 1/3 teaspoon salt
- 1/4 teaspoon cayenne pepper

Directions:

1. Switch on the oven, then set it to 375 °F and let it preheat.

2. Meanwhile, place onion, chickpeas, quinoa into a food processor, and then pulse little chunky mixture comes together.
3. Add water, salt, and cayenne pepper, and then pulse until the dough comes together.
4. Then tip the mixture into a medium bowl, cover it with its lid and then let it rest in the refrigerator for 15 minutes.
5. Shape the mixture into two patties, place them on a baking sheet lined with parchment paper and then bake for 20 minutes, turning halfway.
6. Then switch on the broiler and continue cooking for 2 minutes per side until golden brown.
7. You can serve the patties with tahini cream and salad.

Nutrition: Calories: 315.4, Fat: 9.4 g, Protein: 10.1 g, Carbs: 47.7 g, Fiber: 5.8 g.

Day 5

17. Breakfast: Raspberry, Peach, and Walnuts Smoothie

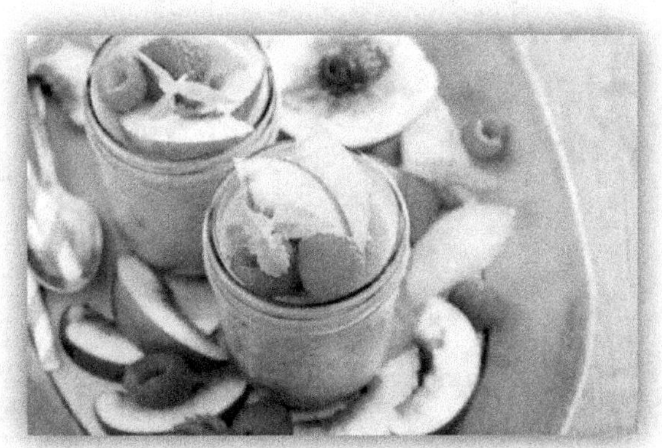

> **Preparation time:** 5 minutes
> **Servings:** 2

Ingredients:

- ½ of peach
- ½ cup raspberries
- 1 ½ tablespoons walnuts
- 2 tablespoons agave syrup
- ½ tablespoon Bromide Plus Powder
- 2 cups spring water

Directions:

1. Plug in a high-speed food processor or blender and add all the ingredients to its jar and pulse for 40 to 60 seconds until smooth.
2. Divide the drink between two glasses and then serve.

Nutrition: Calories: 165, g Fat: 0.3 g, Protein: 12 g, Carbs: 18.7 g, Fiber: 2.5 g.

18. Lunch: Wild Rice and Lentils Bowl

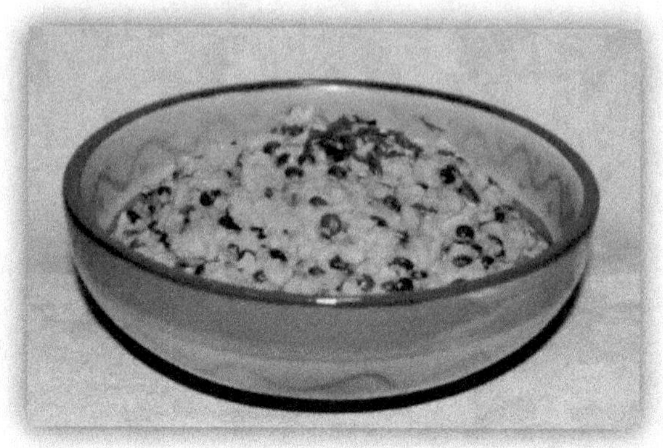

- ➢ **Preparation time:** 10 minutes
- ➢ **Cooking time:** 45 minutes
- ➢ **Servings:** 4

Ingredients:

For the rice

- 2 cups raw wild rice
- 4 cups of spring water
- ½ teaspoon whole sea salt
- 2 bay leaves

For lentils

- 2 cups black lentils
- 1 ¾ cups coconut milk, unsweetened
- 2 cups vegetable broth
- 1 teaspoon dried thyme
- 1 teaspoon dried paprika
- ½ medium onion, peeled
- 1 tablespoon minced garlic
- Parsley for garnish
- 3 tablespoons coconut oil

- 1 teaspoon sea salt
- - ½ teaspoon ground black pepper

Directions:
1. Prepare the rice: take a medium pot, place it over medium-high heat, pour in the water, add the bay leaf and salt.
2. Bring the water to a boil, then change the heat to medium, add the rice and cook for 30-45 minutes or more until tender.
3. When done, remove bay leaves from rice, drain if any water remains in the pot, remove from heat and mash with a fork. Set aside until needed.
4. While the rice is boiling, prepare the lentils: take a large pot, place it over medium-high heat and when hot, add the onion and cook for 5 minutes or until blanched.
5. Add the garlic, cook for 2 minutes until fragrant and golden brown, then add the remaining lentil ingredients and stir until blended.
6. Bring the lentils to a boil, lower the heat and simmer the lentils for 20 minutes until tender, keeping the pot covered.
7. When done, remove the pot from the heat and set aside.
8. Assemble the bowl: divide the rice evenly among four bowls and then add the lentils, adding the parsley.
9. Serve straight away.

Nutrition: Calories: 224, Fat: 1,2. g, Protein: 12,5 g, Carbs: 42,6 g, Fiber: 5.1 g.

19. Snack: Respiratory Power Boost

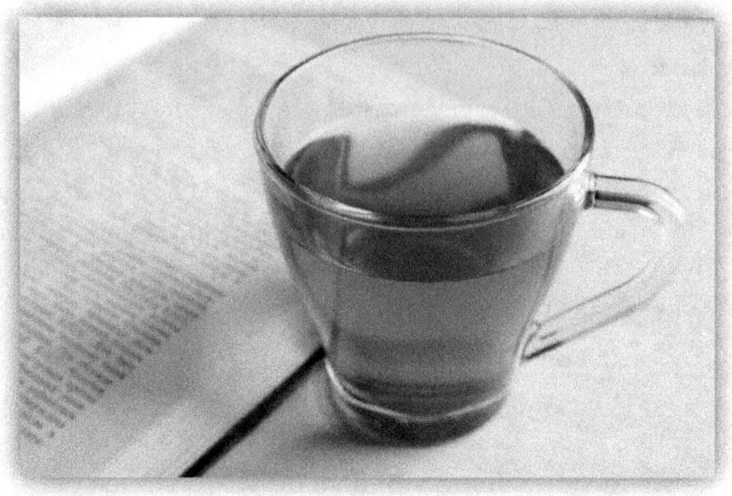

- ➢ **Preparation time:** 5 minutes
- ➢ **Cooking time:** 10 minutes
- ➢ **Servings:** 1

Ingredients:

- 1 teaspoon Guaco herb
- 1 teaspoon Mullein
- 1 cup spring water

Directions:

1. Boil guaco herb and mullein in a tea kettle within 10 minutes. Remove to cool within 10 minutes and serve.

20. Dinner: Roasted Vegetable and St. John's Wort Salad

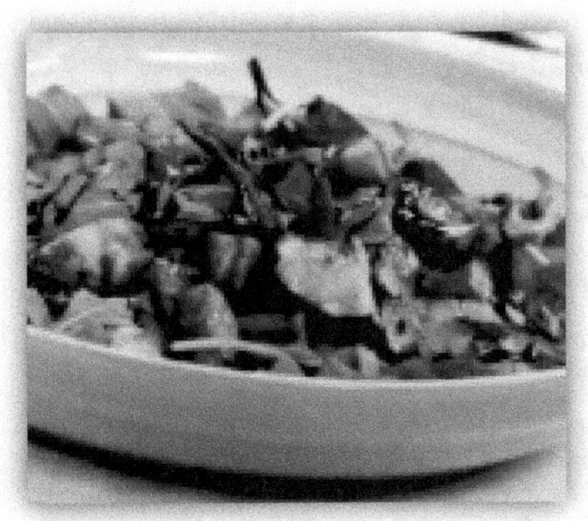

- ➢ **Preparation time:** 15 minutes
- ➢ **Cooking time:** 30 minutes
- ➢ **Servings:** 2

Ingredients:

- 3 tablespoons olive oil
- 1 tablespoon maple syrup
- 1 tablespoon apple cider vinegar
- 1/2 teaspoon sea salt
- 1 tablespoon olive oil
- 4 medium zucchini
- 1 red bell pepper
- 1 red onion, sliced
- 1 fennel, sliced
- 1 teaspoon whole sea salt
- 3 cups beet and spinach leaves
- 2 tablespoons of St. John's wort flowers, dried
- 1 cup arugula

Directions:

1. or the dressing, mix the first 4 ingredients and set aside. Pour all the other ingredients into the olive oil (apart from the St. John's wort leaves and flowers) and place in a previously oiled baking dish.
2. Roast in a preheated oven at 200° for 15 minutes, until the vegetables are tender and a little toasted. Cool to room temperature. Stir in cooled vegetables and fresh leaves.
3. Scatter over the dried flowers and top with the previously prepared dressing.
4. Serve straight away.

Nutrition: Calories: 109, Fat: 9 g, Protein: 7.3 g, Carbs: 24.2 g, Fiber: 6.3 g.

Day 6

---

21. Breakfast: Kamut Porridge with Dates

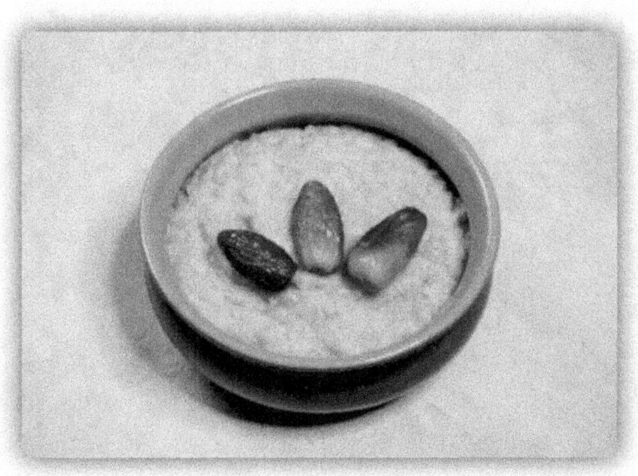

- ➢ Preparation time: 5 minutes
- ➢ Cooking time: 15 minutes
- ➢ Portions: 2

Ingredients:

- 1 cup dates, pitted, chopped
- 1 cup Kamut flakes
- 1/8 teaspoon salt
- 2 cups spring water
- Dates for decoration

Directions:

1. Soak the Kamut flakes in water overnight in a small saucepan.

2. The next morning, add the salt and cook over medium heat for about 10 minutes, stirring constantly;
3. Allow the water to dry, add the dates, stir again and pour into two bowls;
4. If desired, garnish with two dates and serve.

NUTRITION: Calories: 132 Fats: 1 g Protein: 0.3 g Carbohydrates: 30.2 g Fiber: 2

22. Lunch: "Noodles" with Avocado Sauce

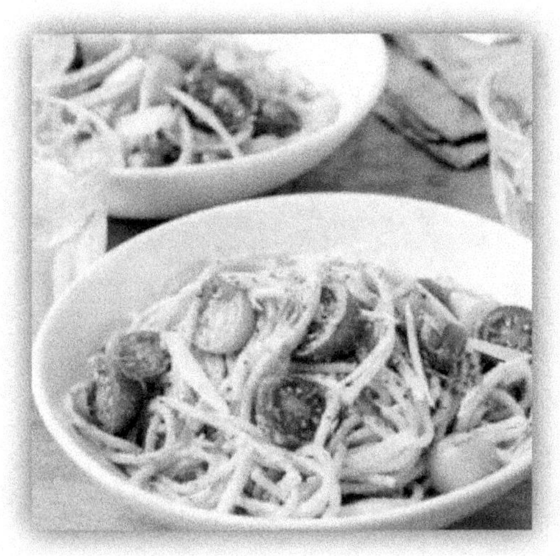

- ➢ **Preparation time:** 30 minutes
- ➢ **Cooking time:** 45 minutes
- ➢ **Servings:** 2

Ingredients:

- 2 large zucchini
- ½ cup walnuts
- 2 cups basil
- 2 avocados
- 4 teaspoons of lime juice
- 2 sliced cherry tomatoes
- Whole grain sea salt to taste
- ½ cup water

Directions:

1. Use a spiralizer to prepare the zucchini noodles.
2. Blend all other ingredients until creamy.
3. Assemble the noodles and avocado sauce in a bowl. Serve and enjoy.

Nutrition: Calories: 26 Fats: 13.5g Carbohydrates: 7.6g Fiber: 3.8g Protein: 4.3g.

23. Snack: Cucumber and Watermelon Detox Smoothie

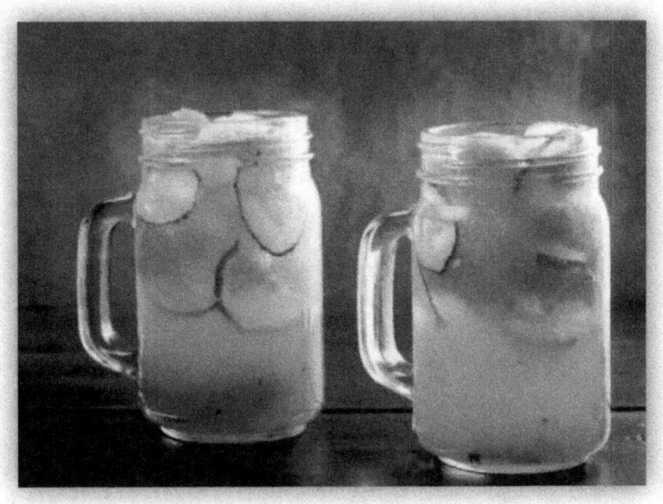

> **Preparation time:** 5 minutes
> **Servings:** 2

Ingredients:

- 1 cucumber
- 1 lime
- 1 cup watermelon, cubed
- ½ cup spring water

Directions:

1. Blend all ingredients in a high-speed blender.
2. Squeeze the lime and add it to the smoothie.
3. Decorate with thin cucumber leaves and then serve.

Nutrition: Calories: 69, Fat; 0 g, Protein: 3 g, Carbs: 48 g, Fiber: 5.4 g.

24. Dinner: Roasted Cauliflower and Walnuts

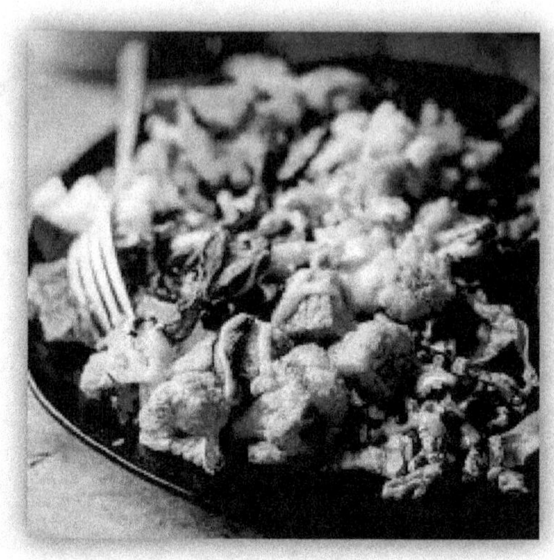

> ➤ **Preparation time:** 15 minutes
> ➤ **Cooking time:** 25 minutes
> ➤ **Servings:** 2

Ingredients:

- 3 cups cauliflower florets
- 2 tablespoons avocado oil
- 1/2 teaspoon turmeric, ground
- 1/4 teaspoon salt
- 1 tablespoon water
- 2 tablespoons miso paste
- 1 green leaf lettuce, cut and cleaned
- ½ cup walnuts

Directions:

1. Heat the oven to 350 °F. Pour the oil over the cauliflower, add turmeric, salt, and mix. Spread it on a baking sheet and bake for 26 minutes.

2. Mix the water and miso in a bowl, transfer to the roasted cauliflower and stir.
3. Divide the shredded lettuce between two plates. Add the roasted cauliflower, walnuts, and avocado oil. Serve.

Nutrition: Calories: 322, Fat: 22 g, Protein: 22 g, Carbs: 19 g. Fiber: 8 g.

Day 7

25. Breakfast: Blueberry Spelt Pancakes

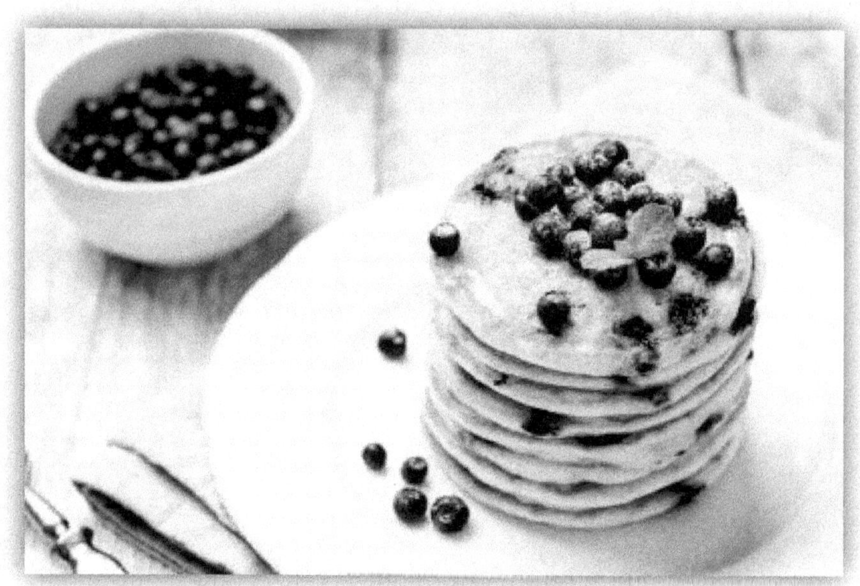

- ➢ **Preparation time:** 10 minutes
- ➢ **Cooking time:** 8 minutes
- ➢ **Servings:** 2

Ingredients:

- 1 cup spelt flour
- ¼ cup blueberries
- ¼ cup agave syrup
- 1/8 teaspoon sea moss
- ½ cup soft-jelly coconut milk
- ¼ cup spring water
- 2 tablespoons grapeseed oil

Directions:

1. Take a large bowl, place flour in it, add agave syrup, 1-tablespoon oil, and sea moss, and then stir until mixed.

2. Whisk in milk and water until smooth batter comes together and then fold in berries.

3. Take a large skillet pan, place it over medium heat, add remaining oil and when hot, ladle batter in it, shape into a pancake and then cook for 2 to 3 minutes per side until golden brown and cooked.

4. Serve straight away.

Nutrition: Calories: 156, Fat: 3.6 g, Protein. 8.4 g, Carbs: 22.8 g, Fiber: 3.3.g.

26. Lunch: Ratatouille and Quinoa Stew

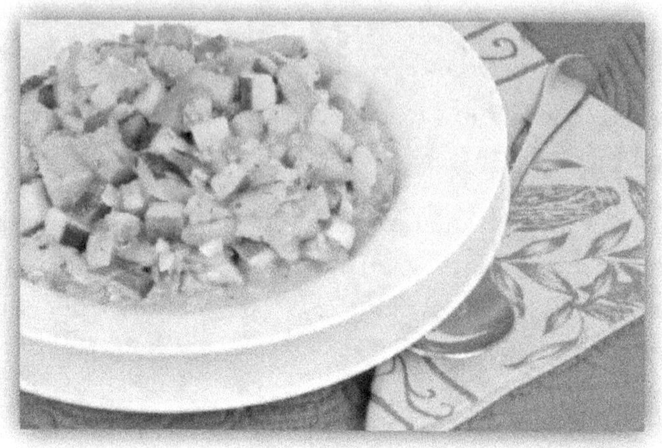

- ➢ **Preparation time:** 5 minutes
- ➢ **Cooking time:** 30 minutes
- ➢ **Servings:** 2

Ingredients:

- 1 ½ cups eggplant, diced.
- 1 ½ cups squash, cut into four and sliced.
- 2 cloves garlic, minced.
- 1 ½ cups chopped onion.
- ½ cup quinoa.
- 6 cups vegetable broth.
- 3 cups crushed tomatoes.
- ¼ cup jarred chiles, chopped.
- 3 bay leaves.
- 1 tablespoon olive oil.
- 1 ½ teaspoons dried thyme leaves.

Directions:

1. Preheat a Dutch oven over medium heat. Add the eggplant, onions, garlic, and zucchini. Bake for about 2 minutes.

2. Add the quinoa, bay leaf, and thyme and sauté for about 8 minutes more. Add the vegetable stock, tomatoes, and peppers. Bring to a boil.
3. Cover, set heat to low, and let cook for another 20 minutes. Remove from heat. Serve and enjoy!

Nutrition: Calories: 90, Fat: 2 g, Protein: 9 g, Carbs: 16 g, Fiber: 4 g.

27. Snack: Invigorating Sea Moss Pudding

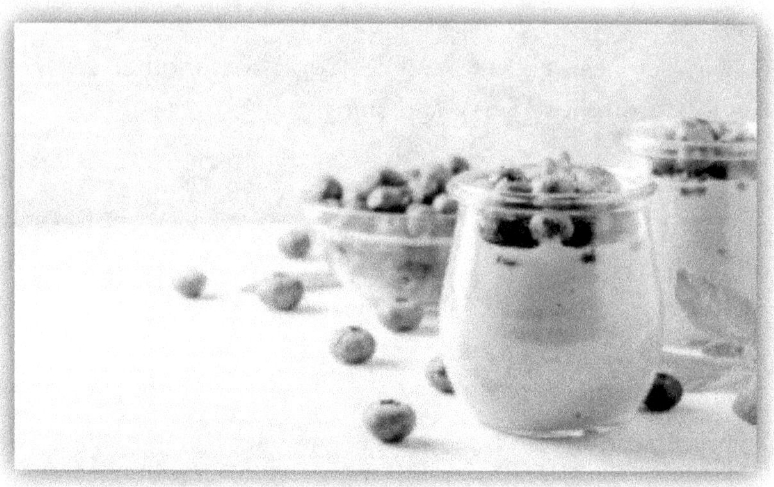

> **Preparation time:** 5 minutes
> **Servings:** 2

Ingredients:

- 2 burro bananas, peeled
- 2 cups blueberries
- 6 tablespoons of sea moss gel
- ½ cup spring water

Directions:

1. Plug in a high-speed food processor or blender and add all the ingredients in its jar except for water.
2. Cover the blender jar with its lid, pulse until smooth, and then slowly blend in water until thickened to the desired level.
3. Serve straight away.

Nutrition: Calories: 97.8 g, Fat: 0.5 g, Protein: 0.7 g, Carbs: 23.4 g, Fiber: 2.8 g.

28. Dinner: Teff Grain Burger

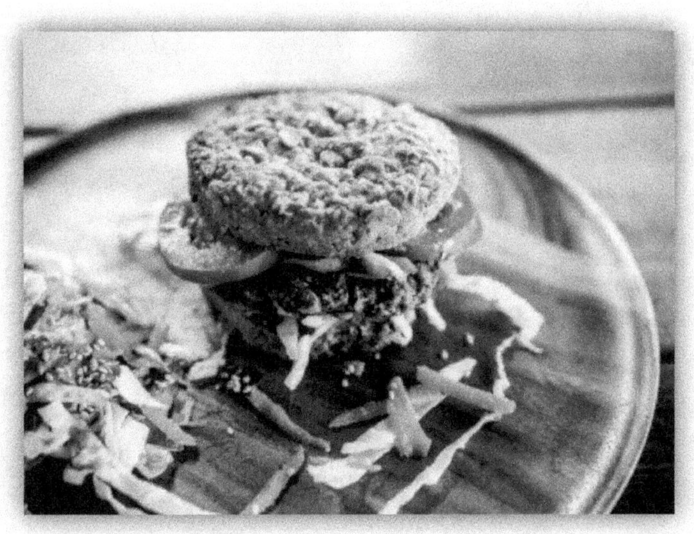

> **Preparation time:** 10 minutes
> **Cooking time:** 8 minutes
> **Servings:** 2

Ingredients:

- 2 teff grain buns
- 2/3 cup chickpea flour
- 2/3 cup sliced cooked squash
- 2/3 cup sliced lettuce
- 2 tablespoons diced onion
- 2 tablespoons cherry tomatoes
- 1½ tablespoons diced red bell pepper

- ½ teaspoon dill
- 2/5 teaspoon salt
- ½ teaspoon oregano
- 5/8 teaspoon cayenne pepper
- ½ teaspoon basil
- 1 tablespoon grape seed oil

Directions:

1. Prepare a medium-sized skillet, add the oil and heat over medium heat;
2. Make sure it heats up well before adding the onions and bell pepper. Then, let it cook on low heat for 5 minutes;
3. Meanwhile, pour the vegetables into a medium-sized bowl, add all the other ingredients and mix, then form into balls and shape into burgers.
4. Place them in the hot skillet, cook for 4 minutes until golden brown on both sides.
5. Remove from heat, place all in buns and serve immediately with cherry tomatoes, squash and salad.

Nutrition: Calories: 122, Fat: 4.1 g, 4.2 g Protein, 4.2 g, Carbs: 16.6 g, Fiber: 2.6 g.

CONCLUSION

Now, you have learned more about Dr. Sebi's alkaline diet. You know how to prepare your meals, the meal plan for each day of the week, and what foods you should eat. In this book, we talked about how alkaline eating can help reverse disease and weight loss. In addition, about why alkaline food is so healthy for us and how it can reverse disease in people when combined with proper lifestyle.

However, that's not all! You learned why alkaline food is good for you and your diet. You now have an understanding of what the different types of acidity are and which ones will make your body function worse in any type of situation.

Dr. Sebi's diet may have many restrictions on what to eat and what not to eat. However, you will find foods that taste great and can be incorporated into your everyday meals and snacks.

This book wants to empower people through knowledge, so that they can make informed decisions on how to eat for the rest of your life. Try out the alkaline diet for at least 30 days and see if it works for you. If, after 30 days, you do not see a difference in your health or weight, then stop the alkaline diet and go back to eating how you were before… Want to bet it won't happen?

Through this book, you have learned about the foods that can be your friend. By following this type of diet, your body will function at its best and most likely, increasing its performance.

We also get to know more about the functions and miraculous powers of herbs that Dr. Sebi approved. By incorporating them into your alkaline anti-inflammatory diet, they can really help cleanse your body in a deep and lasting way.

People may have a hard time adjusting and changing their eating habits, but all you need to get started is organization and… a little discipline.

In the end, following Dr. Sebi's diet will be worth it. Why? Because you're doing something great for your body! You're giving it the proper nutrients it needs to stay healthy in the long term.

You can easily start with the detox week I've provided in this book and begin your journey. Of course, you should always consult your doctor before following any diet and exercise plan.

I wish you the best.

Tasha Dixon.

Download now completely for free your bonus: "A 7-day alkaline plan, to detox your liver and intestine," by clicking on this link: https://rebrand.ly/ikigaipublishing (if you have the kindle version) or by scanning this QR code with your mobile phone, (if you have the paperback version), and then follow the instructions to download the free meal plan with recipes and colored photos.